"This unusual book bridges the unhappy divide between pro-life and social-justice approaches to the U.S. healthcare system. Camosy's provocative conclusions should stimulate all to think hard about the real, practical effects of their moral positions. At a deeper level, Camosy proposes a radical and needed defense of the sociality of the person and the interdependence of individual interests and the common good."

— LISA SOWLE CAHILL
Boston College

"In this crisply argued and tightly focused book, Charles Camosy strips away contemporary evasions of the rationing that is already taking place in American medicine. By asking what Christians owe to 'imperiled' rather than 'disabled' newborns, he is able to make powerful links between ancient Christian views and today's debates about health care rationing for fragile newborns. Perhaps most importantly, Camosy goes far beyond most medical ethics in insisting that these questions be faced as part of a larger moral analysis of the amazing inequalities that characterize contemporary health care in the United States."

— BRIAN BROCK
University of Aberdeen

"Camosy's bracing argument is honest, clear, informed, and pervasively Catholic in its sources, yet it will be persuasive to many outside that tradition as well."

— JAMES C. PETERSON
McMaster University

"This book is an excellent example of how Roman Catholic theology can boldly engage society at large. Camosy discusses neonatal intensive care in great detail and shows how we unjustly ration this form of care in the United States. He goes on to propose how our society might do this more justly and also suggests how Christians might practice hospitality toward those who have been denied care."

— STEPHEN E. LAMMERS
Lafayette College

# TOO EXPENSIVE TO TREAT?

*Finitude, Tragedy, and the Neonatal ICU*

Charles C. Camosy

WILLIAM B. EERDMANS PUBLISHING COMPANY
GRAND RAPIDS, MICHIGAN / CAMBRIDGE, U.K.

Published 2010 by
Wm. B. Eerdmans Publishing Co.
2140 Oak Industrial Drive N.E., Grand Rapids, Michigan 49505 /
P.O. Box 163, Cambridge CB3 9PU U.K.

Printed in the United States of America

15 14 13 12 11 10     7 6 5 4 3 2 1

**Library of Congress Cataloging-in-Publication Data**

Camosy, Charles Christopher.
Too expensive to treat?: finitude, tragedy, and the neonatal ICU / Charles C. Camosy.
p.     cm.
Includes bibliographical references (p.     ).
ISBN 978-0-8028-6529-8 (pbk.: alk. paper)
1. Neonatal intensive care — Moral and ethical aspects. I. Title.
RJ253.5.C36   2010
174.2'9892'01 — dc22

2010040495

www.eerdmans.com

# Contents

# Acknowledgments

This book would not have been possible without the support, insight, and consistent friendly pushes from my mentors at the University of Notre Dame. In particular I want to thank Todd Whitmore, Jerry McKenny, and of course Maura Ryan. I'd also like to thank the Center for the Study of Bioethics at the Medical College of Wisconsin for giving me a year visiting fellowship which included an invaluable chance to round with neonatal intensive care staff at Children's Hospital of Milwaukee. Special consideration goes to Steve Leuthner, M.D., who walked me through the complexities of neonatology and offered many helpful comments on multiple drafts of this manuscript. Robert White, M.D., also offered his expertise in neonatology at several points in the research and writing process. The research grant offered by the Nanovic Institute for European Studies at Notre Dame to visit NICUs in the Netherlands was an especially nice boost to my research — and I owe Dr. Carlo Leget much for his hosting me while there. A faculty research grant from Fordham University's office of sponsored programs was also an important support for this project. I was very fortunate to have two thorough and insightful edits done by Katie Ball-Boruff and Joel Warden — and am grateful for Monica Pierce's work on the index.

Special thanks of course go to Jon Pott and Eerdmans Publishing for their support of, and insights into, this project. A portion of the first chapter was drawn from a previously published article, "Common Ground on Surgical Abortion? — Engaging Peter Singer on the Moral Status of Potential Persons," *Journal of Medicine and Philosophy* 33, no. 6

(2008): 577-93. I am grateful for the journal's permission to use some of the material for this book.

Finally, let me acknowledge and thank several people who started me on the path I am currently walking. Brad Malkovsky: his inspiration convinced me to do doctoral work. Jean Porter: her class and mentorship helped me to decide that I wanted to do ethics. And finally my parents and grandparents: thank you for your past, current, and future support. I want to make special mention of support which came from my mother — which went far beyond her sharing with me a love for theology and for our church.

# Introduction

This book is about moral tragedy. Though I will focus most of my attention on how it plays out in the context of neonatal medicine, there surely is a similar kind of tragedy in numerous other medical contexts about which a different book could be written. Such tragedy is the inevitable result of two universal aspects of the human condition:

1. We have virtually unlimited health care needs.[1]
2. We have limited health care resources.[2]

We cannot escape the tragedy of being unable to provide for everyone's health care needs any more than we can escape our finite human nature and resources. We are simply destined, based on who we are and the situation in which we find ourselves, to live with this hard and disconcerting truth.

However, though we must live in this *tragic* situation, we need not live in an *unjust* situation. The former is unavoidable, but the latter is a result of immoral choices and social structures. As this book goes to press, the unjust health care system of the United States has once again sparked a heated national debate about precisely what reforms should take place to make it more just. Many of those against expanding our

1. As the *Onion* helpfully reminds us, the "World Death Rate Is Holding Steady at 100%." See http://www.theonion.com/articles/world-death-rate-holding-steady-at-100-percent,1670/ (accessed June 27, 2009).

2. This is especially true if we see the good of health care in the context of a multitude of goods necessary for flourishing.

already significant public option for health insurance cry out against the "rationing" that would be done. Even the Obama administration and others pushing for precisely this kind of expansion claim that "no one is talking about rationing."[3] But what neither side seems to realize, or at least is willing to admit, is that *we are already rationing* and we will never *not* be rationing. In the system used for the past few generations, and the one in place as this book goes to press, we have decided to ration public health care monies with preference for the impoverished (Medicaid) and the retired (Medicare). Most others get their insurance through a tax-free medical benefit from their employers. Of course, our rationing plan simply bites the bullet on several dozen million persons who do not have any health insurance at all. And even in the event that a reformed U.S. health care system ends up covering many of these individuals (all the plans being currently debated still leave many millions uninsured), the rationing questions will not go away. Indeed, they will get more pronounced. Take the National Health Service of the United Kingdom; though it "covers" everyone, because the British understand better than most Americans that they do not have enough resources to meet every single health care need, they are quite explicit about their need to ration care. One could bring up any number of examples in support of this claim, but a dramatic one that has special import for this book is of a physician telling a U.K. woman in September 2009 that "it was against the rules to save her premature baby."[4]

And then there is the rationing within the rationing. Insurance companies certainly do not pay for every medical need of their customers — nor could they. What sorts of treatments are covered and how much of the bill will be paid are negotiated with health care providers. Often they will use what governments at the state and federal levels treat and reimburse with Medicaid and Medicare as a baseline from which to negotiate. These U.S. government programs are quite explicit

3. Fred Lucas, "White House Vows No Rationing in Health Care Reform Package," CNS News, June 3, 2009; http://www.cnsnews.com/Public/Content/article.aspx?RsrcID =49010 (accessed June 27, 2009).

4. Vanessa Allen and Andrew Levy, "Doctors Told Me It Was against the Rules to Save My Premature Baby," *MailOnline*, September 10, 2009; http://www.dailymail.co.uk/news/article-1211950/Premature-baby-left-die-doctors-mother-gives-birth-just-days-22-week-care-limit.html (accessed October 30, 2009). The "rules" mentioned here were set by the well-respected Nuffield Bioethics Council.

in their rationing of resources.[5] However, when we continue to refuse to admit as a culture what we are doing, we refuse to challenge the unjust way the de facto rationing is taking place. This is especially true if, as the leadership of the Roman Catholic Church and many others argue,[6] all persons have a right to have their fundamental health care needs met. Instead of a rationing aimed at meeting this duty of justice, we currently have a market- and politics-driven rationing that favors diseases of the rich, the politically powerful, the publicly sympathetic, and those without preexisting conditions or predispositions to disease. This leaves millions without any insurance at all — and many millions more dramatically underinsured.

So while it is true that we will never escape the unavoidable tragedy of forced health care rationing, it is also true that we need not stand by while it is unjustly implemented. Though in this book I will focus on the context of neonatal intensive care, in many other contexts of medicine there is similar need for investigation, criticism, and reform. This book is but a single step in what will hopefully be a broad, multi-pronged movement in health care reform: (1) an honest acknowledgment of the inescapable need to ration resources, and (2) a rationing that has justice and the common good — rather than politics and ability to pay — as its guiding principles.

## The Context of Neonatal Intensive Care

Even if one only intermittently follows world news, it is virtually impossible to avoid the attention ethical issues surrounding newborn infants receive. For instance, a much anticipated report from the Nuffield

5. As the United States prepares to expand Medicaid to cover many who are currently uninsured, we will likely see this kind of rationing up front and center in our public discourse.

6. I write this book from the perspective of a Roman Catholic ethicist, but I hope the theological principles invoked in the text are sufficiently "thin" that readers can engage them without necessarily accepting the "thicker" theological claims of the Catholic Church. Indeed, the central ethical principles invoked in this book — the right to health care, a relational anthropology, the moral status of the newborn infant, a distinction between beneficial and burdensome treatment, and the priority of the common good — are generally accepted by several faiths and many with no explicit faith tradition.

Council on Bioethics[7] has called for a uniform policy under which newborns born under twenty-two weeks gestation are to be refused treatment regardless of prognosis.[8] Almost on cue, a record was set in Florida when, remarkably, a baby of less than twenty-two weeks gestation survived NICU (neonatal intensive care unit) treatment with a good prognosis.[9] The Church of England's Bishop Butler created headlines all over the world by arguing in January 2007 that when considering whether or not to treat imperiled newborns, "The principle of justice inevitably means that the potential cost of treatment itself, the longer term costs of health care and education and opportunity cost to the NHS [National Health Service] in terms of saving other lives have to be considered."

The media's coverage of the issues surrounding the medical treatment of imperiled newborns, perhaps not surprisingly, leaves much to be desired. For instance, a typical headline in response to the above "shock" claim of the bishop was "Outrage as Church Calls for Severely Disabled Babies to Be *Killed* at Birth" (emphasis added).[10] But of course, he never made this claim; indeed, the Christian moral tradition generally prohibits aiming at death as part of one's intentional action or omission. Rather, as we will see in some detail, the call was for the refusal of a treatment deemed too burdensome. In addition, the article's author claimed that this flew in the face of the history of Christian thought, which "has long argued that life should [be] preserved at all costs." Though the issues surrounding withholding or withdrawing life-sustaining treatment are complex (and, admittedly, the diverse

7. An internationally respected group of clinicians, lawyers, philosophers, scientists, and theologians established by the Trustees of the Nuffield Foundation (U.K.) in 1991 to identify, examine, and report on the ethical questions raised by recent advances in biological and medical research. The report in question came out November 16, 2006, and can be found at www.nuffieldbioethics.org/go/ourwork/neonatal/introduction.

8. Jeremy Laurance, "Critics Condemn 23-Week Premature Baby Ban," *Independent*, November 16, 2006; http://news.independent.co.uk/uk/health_medical/article1987614 .ece (accessed January 27, 2007).

9. Aida Edemariam, "Against All Odds," *Guardian*, February 21, 2007; http:// www.guardian.co.uk/medicine/story/0,,2017772,00.html (accessed September 14, 2007).

10. Neal Sears, "Outrage as Church Calls for Severely Disabled Babies to Be Killed at Birth," *MailOnline*, November 12, 2006; http://www.dailymail.co.uk/pages/live/ articles/news/news.html?in_article_id=416003&in_page_id=1770 (accessed January 27, 2007).

Christian community today has differing opinions on these matters), the last five centuries of Roman Catholic teaching directly contradict this common misconception.[11] If those whose job it is to professionally cover these stories can make these kinds of fundamental errors, it is not surprising that others are often confused by these issues as well. The technological advances in neonatology over the last forty years have produced some of the most complex and multifaceted dilemmas in all of medicine. As Michael Panicola has pointed out, "Nowhere is this [complexity] more evident than in cases involving critically ill newborns."[12] Neonatal patients, unlike more traditional ones, "have never expressed either explicitly or implicitly what values they want to pursue in life, what condition they find too burdensome, or what treatments they consider contrary to their best interests. Consequently, proxy decision makers must make value-laden assumptions for them before deciding whether to initiate or continue life-sustaining treatment."[13]

Though still quite complex, the issues surrounding the treatment of newborns were not always so connected with technology — and indeed go back to ancient times. Soranus of Ephesus, a second-century Greek physician, gave midwives a practical handbook for newborn infants that were "worth rearing" or "suited by nature for rearing."[14] In addition to receiving systematic treatment in the ancient pagan world, these issues were a focus, from the beginning, for the very first Christian traditions. The *Didache*, Justin Martyr's *First Apology*, and Athenagoras's *Plea* are all at pains to critically engage pagan practices toward imperiled newborns. Chapter 1 will go into more detail regarding these historical manifestations of the ethical issues central to this book, but here we note that though many times infants were killed or left to die due to poverty and other social factors, the point of contention was often the *moral status* of the newly born — and especially of newborn females. The early Christian traditions generally spoke up in favor of the moral status and treatment of imperiled newborns, and many acted on

11. Indeed, this book will show in some detail just how mistaken this claim is.

12. Michael R. Panicola, "Quality of Life and the Critically Ill Newborn: Life and Death Decision Making in the Neonatal Context" (Ph.D. diss., Saint Louis University, 2000), 2.

13. Panicola, "Quality of Life," 56.

14. Soranus, *Gynecology*, vol. 3 (Baltimore: Johns Hopkins University Press, 1956), 258.

this conviction by saving "exposed" infants who had been left to die or to be picked up for the slave trade or forced prostitution.

Of central interest to this book, however, is the layer of complexity added by the technological shift of our modern era — an era that began in earnest when premature infants with respiratory distress syndrome started to survive due to new technical innovations in the mid to late twentieth century. Millions of infants survived who otherwise would have died — and even more have had their lives improved through treatment. As Panicola notes, "Not long ago few newborns weighing less than 750 grams were treated because treatment was considered futile. Today, however, newborns weighing at least 500 grams and newborns born at 24 weeks gestation routinely receive intensive care in the United States."[15]

The results of this shift are open to interpretation. While many have been saved that otherwise would have died, "An alarming number of newborns saved by neonatal medicine experience significant medical problems, and must often contend with mental and physical impairments, multiple surgeries, chronic pain and suffering, lengthy dependence on ventilators, prolonged hospitalization, extensive rehabilitation, and special education. . . . Families often experience significant financial burdens and society is drained of previous healthcare resources in caring for sick newborns, especially those born extremely small and immature."[16] Following the technological advances that produced the above outcomes, concerns about the quality of life for imperiled newborns began to come to the fore. In the last several years we have been forced to "accept the responsibility for the power we have obtained and ask the frightening question, 'What kind of life are we saving?'"[17]

In attempting to answer the above question, a "quality of life" model of decision making has been advocated by certain ethicists and physicians. What exactly counts as quality of life, however, is certainly a disputed question. One way to think about it, Panicola notes, is how proxy decision makers evaluate the benefits and burdens of various life-sustaining interventions in light of the overall medical condition

---

15. Panicola, "Quality of Life," 18.
16. Panicola, "Quality of Life," 20-21.
17. Panicola, "Quality of Life," 3.

of critically ill newborns. For instance, one might weigh the burden of a medical treatment that involves extreme pain and a very long hospital stay versus the benefit of a chance at continued life. But even if one accepts this quality of life model at a general level (and many do not), how one defines "benefit" and "burden" can be contentious.[18] Some claim that these concepts are too vague or ambiguous to be applied with any consistency in neonatal decision making. Do they refer only to something about the medical realities of the child herself? What about psychological or spiritual realities? Can the best interests of a newborn include how others are affected by her care? What or who counts as "others"? Family? Community? A globalized world?

Panicola helpfully distinguishes between three different submodels of the quality of life approach. The "individual quality of life" model centers explicitly on the newborn. The "relational quality of life" model focuses on the newborn's ability to pursue life's goals, understood as material, moral, and spiritual values that transcend physical life. The "social quality of life" model centers on the newborn specifically in her familial and social context. This latter model appears to be the only one able to give social factors the weight they deserve — especially in light of an important point made by the John B. Francis Chair in Bioethics at the Center for Practical Bioethics in Kansas City, John Lantos: "Neonatal intensive care has become some of the most expensive in pediatrics. Before the advent of neonatology, it was inconceivable to spend hundreds of thousands of dollars to save a baby's life. Today it has become routine and routinely disturbing. . . . Furthermore, because of the idiosyncrasies of healthcare financing rules, NICUs have become profit centers for many U.S. companies."[19] In addition, while it might be natural to think that neonatal bioethics would focus on "a frontier filled with cataclysmic struggles fought by heroic crusaders against implacable biological constraints, with tiny human infants as the battleground," mostly it does not. "Instead, today's NICU is a surprisingly mundane place that runs like a happy factory, churning out healthy baby after healthy baby, with mostly routine efforts by highly trained professionals. Undeniably, dramatic and morally charged

---

18. Panicola, "Quality of Life," 4.

19. John D. Lantos and William Meadow, *Neonatal Bioethics: The Moral Challenges of Medical Innovation* (Baltimore: Johns Hopkins University Press, 2006), 6.

events occur, including agonizing decisions about whether to continue treatment; however, they do not occur very often."[20]

## The Argument

I will argue, then, that the most important issues of neonatal bioethics are primarily *social* in nature — and therefore the social quality of life model is the most helpful for decision making in this context. I will also argue, however, that the current debate surrounding this model has important shortcomings. First, if full moral status is affirmed for imperiled newborns — that is, we consider them to be full persons like any other (as most do) — then this is oftentimes a "conversation stopper," as if there were no further questions to ask. This book's argument will begin by claiming, along with the broadly Christian moral traditions, that intending the death of an innocent person is not permitted. But this still leaves a host of questions to answer about treatment and care. Second, those who argue for a "strong" version of the social quality of life model (a version that sees social factors like distribution of resources as *primary* considerations in the benefit/burden calculation Panicola mentions above) tend to connect it to less than full moral status for imperiled newborns. Third, those who argue for a "weak" version of this model (a version that sees social factors as *merely secondary* considerations in the benefit/burden calculation for a particular treatment), while affirming full moral status for imperiled newborns, generally do not appreciate the full weight that social considerations should play in whether or not to treat. There appear, then, to be three "families" of approaches to the social quality of life model:

1. It is a good model. Many, most, or all infants have something less than full moral status and therefore are not persons. Given a lack of medical resources for those who are persons, those human infants with less than full moral status can or should be denied treatment based on broad social factors, and such factors have primary importance.
2. It is a bad model. Human infants are persons, and as such have in-

20. Lantos and Meadow, *Neonatal Bioethics*, 10.

trinsic dignity that cannot (theory-based objection) or should not (practice-based objection) be overridden by treatment decisions made on the basis of social considerations such as cost or resource allocation.

3. It is a good model. Though many, most, or all human infants have full moral status, social factors can and should play a role in the treatment decision-making process. But rather than being primary, they are secondary, balance-tipping factors — often focusing on the narrowly considered "best interests" of the infant.

The first three chapters of the book will detail and respond to each position above in turn. I will argue that the first approach mistakenly claims that imperiled newborns do not have full moral status. The second, insofar as it has Christian commitments in this area (and the thinkers that I address here will), misunderstands the role the social factors have played in the broadly Christian tradition in distinguishing between ordinary and extraordinary means and also does not appreciate the human person's identity as essentially intrinsically social. The third misses the full weight that social factors should play in determining whether or not a treatment is extraordinary — something seen clearly when the principles and theological anthropology of Catholic social teaching are brought to bear.

But in the final chapter I will argue for a fourth approach:

4. It is a good model. Though all human infants have full moral status, if one accepts Catholic social teaching's principles of theological anthropology, universal destination of goods, and a preferential option for the poor, broad social factors have more than secondary importance when it comes to treatment of imperiled newborns.

I will also claim that while consideration of the moral status of newborns should be a first and foundational step, it should be seen as distinctive from formal discussion of the social quality of life model. Once separated from the issue of the moral status, the other two approaches to the social quality of life model will be considered in light of (1) Roman Catholic teaching on ordinary and extraordinary means and (2) Catholic social teaching — both of which have been largely absorbed into secular medicine and ethics. My central thesis is that though we must never compromise on the fundamental truth that all newly born human infants (even those with the most serious diseases and challenges) are persons with full moral status, whether particular treatments are beneficial or burdensome cannot be seen apart from consideration of complex social questions about distribution of resources.[21] In other words, each and every newborn baby counts just as much as a more mature human person — but not *more*. Care must be taken to ration resources justly and in due proportion with the common good.

## Complications and Objections

My experience has been that many find the above argument understandably distasteful and even shocking. They often react by saying, "We cannot put a price on life" and "Abstract arguments fail to respect the power of personal stories and experience." And, truth be told, I have much sympathy for these points of view. Christine Gleason, M.D., chief of neonatology at Seattle Children's Hospital, recently wrote a book that made the latter point about personal experience quite well. Consider this moving passage in which Dr. Gleason describes one of her past patients, Patrick, who beat the odds and was the first baby his size to survive at her hospital. Clearly, he was a fighter.

> Nearly three months after he was plucked from his mother's womb to save her life, Patrick was ready to go home. He weighed three and a half pounds, less than most preemies do at the time of discharge, but he remembered to breathe; he could take all of his feedings through a bottle; his penis had grown enough that he was circumcised. . . . He had graduated to the bassinet, just like the ones that full-term babies go into after they're born, and he looked so tiny in it. I picked him up and carried him over to a nearby rocking chair and sat down with him. As I rocked him slowly back and forth, our eyes met and he stared at me intently. It was as though there was a brief moment of recognition. . . . These were the same eyes that had

---

21. The book will limit itself to the question of how resources should be distributed on a state or national level. Factoring in social questions about global health inequities would be exponentially more complex — but would, I think, do nothing but make the central thesis of the book that much stronger.

looked directly at me a couple of months ago, eyes that made me hope that this baby was a "keeper" despite his unbelievably small size.[22]

It is difficult not to have a strong emotional reaction to this story. How could one even think about some kind of abstract argument that might deny treatment to someone like Patrick?

But one must always put a personal story in context with other personal stories. Consider one of the stories we will look at in more detail in chapter 3, that of Jerry from Jackson, Tennessee:

> Jerry has muscle spasms in his heart — a condition that requires him to take eight pills every day and to see a cardiologist. He has no income other than $157 per month in food stamps and lives with his parents. When he was dropped from TennCare [Medicaid] he showed up for a cardiologist appointment and was told that his insurance would no longer pay for the visit. "I couldn't pay for the appointment without TennCare coverage," Jerry said, "so I simply didn't see my doctor that day." Even with his discount card, his drugs cost $400 — which he cannot afford. Recently, he has experienced severe pain in his right arm that prevents him from raising it. "I would have liked to go to the doctor for it, but I couldn't afford to," he said. Jerry has tried to get on disability insurance, but his application was denied.

Can we justify spending $30 million on a single NICU patient[23] while millions like Jerry need live-sustaining treatment — and for pennies on the dollar in comparison? If we say no, we are not putting a price on life. We are not saying that Jerry is worth more than Patrick.[24] We are not even saying that such monies, to be justly distributed, need to go

---

22. Christine Gleason, *Almost Home: Stories of Hope and the Human Spirit* (New York: Kaplan Publishing, 2009), 56-57.

23. This refers to the cost of "Baby Sidney's" treatment in Texas, which we will look at in more detail later in the book.

24. Indeed, I am aware that some reading this book may have spent time in the NICU themselves as a baby — or had someone close to them who did. Some might even be NICU professionals. Let me be clear: this book is making no claims about the worth of anyone's life or profession. This is an argument about how to fairly distribute resources when all participants are seen as having equal worth and value.

somewhere other than toward the health care of babies.[25] We are saying rather that just distribution of resources requires us to face difficult choices about how to ration care. We are saying that regardless of whether one is old or young, rich or poor, disabled or not,[26] part of a racial minority or majority, everyone has equal dignity and an equal right to use a proportionate amount of community resources. Unfortunately, in light of our tragic and finite human condition, this means some will not get care from which they could certainly benefit.

Our hyper-autonomous culture finds it difficult to prioritize justice over and against personal freedom, autonomy, and choice in general, but in the above way in particular. Indeed, some try to pretend that medicine can consider only the narrow good of the individual patient in a contextless vacuum — and some even believe that this way of thinking is part of the *very foundations* of medicine.[27] But those who accept a more relational understanding of the human person as offered by Roman Catholic social teaching (and by many secular schools of thought)[28] must be skeptical of this understanding of medicine. Human dignity cannot be seen outside of its social context — and individ-

25. At the end of chapter 4 I argue that many more resources need to be taken from NICU care and distributed in the form of *prenatal* care — which would avoid a significant cause of NICU admission in the first place.

26. I want to also mention here that my argument makes no judgments at all about "quality of life." This is a dangerous road down which to go — especially because the concept itself is so slippery and ill defined. British ethicist and neonatologist John Wyatt, for instance, has shown that those who are not disabled consistently rate the quality of life of the disabled significantly lower than the disabled persons themselves. Wyatt, "End-of-Life Decisions, Duality of Life and the Newborn," *Acta Paediatrica* 96, no. 6 (June 2007). Also, removing or forgoing treatment because a life is "not worth living" is in fact aiming at death — and, at least according to current Roman Catholic teaching, is euthanasia by omission. No, the central argument of this book limits itself to allocation of resources and avoids the thorny and dangerous issue of quality of life altogether.

27. This, however, is called into serious question given the fact that 65 percent of neonatal physicians and 75 percent of neonatal nurses "gave economic costs of intensive and lifelong care as a reason" for thinking that not all infants in the NICU should be saved. Geoffrey Miller, *Extreme Prematurity: Practices, Bioethics, and the Law* (Cambridge and New York: Cambridge University Press, 2007), 38.

28. Though I make my argument in the context of Catholic social teaching, both are aimed at "all people of good will." Indeed, even those suspicious of Catholic moral theology often share the relational anthropology of its social doctrine. Much more will be said about this in chapter 3.

ual rights are always connected to corresponding social duties. One of these duties, surely, is to use resources in due proportion with the common good.

Now, some argue that this kind of move in the context of neonatal intensive care can only be done while simultaneously challenging the full moral status of newborn children. It is to this argument we now turn.

# CHAPTER I

# The Moral Status of Newborn Infants

*If you are delivered of a child [before I come home], if it is a boy keep it, if a girl discard it.*

Hilarion of Alexandria
Letter to his pregnant wife Alis (I B.C.E.)

*What we are saying to the people is have your children, don't kill them. And if you don't want a girl child, leave her to us.*

Renuka Chowdhury
Indian minister of state for woman
and child development (2007 C.E.)

Not every version of the social quality of life model gives social factors the same weight when making treatment decisions. Though there is overlap and gray area, approaches to this model can generally be characterized as either "weak" or "strong." The weak versions tend to see social factors like "just distribution of resources" as valid but secondary considerations when making decisions about treatment of infants in the NICU. Perhaps they should be taken into consideration as a balance-tipping factor when other, more primary factors do not indicate a clear treatment decision, but they themselves should not form the primary basis for a treatment decision. This point of view will be considered in some detail in chapter 3. The strong versions of the model, by contrast, tend to see social factors as *primary* considerations.

However, most, if not all, strong versions come to their conclusions — at least in part — because they also hold that "newborns are not considered equal members of the moral community."[1] H. Tristram Engelhardt Jr., Joseph Fletcher, Earl Shelp, Michael Tooley, and Peter Singer all hold the position that at least some imperiled newborns do not have the same moral status as most other human beings and are not "full persons" in the moral sense of the word.[2] Having this position certainly paves the way for accepting the strong version of the social quality of life model because it seems clear that limited medical resources should certainly be used on persons before nonpersons — and if many millions of people in the United States (with many hundreds of millions more around the world)[3] do not have health insurance, then some newly born human nonpersons should have their treatment forgone in favor of using such resources on actual persons.

The goal of this chapter is to both (1) take seriously the argument that the newborn is a nonperson and (2) call this argument, and its use in support of the strong version of the social quality of life model, into serious question. In doing so, the chapter will first consider some ancient and modern historical highlights that, when seen in combination with cogent arguments, give us good reason to take the question of the moral status of imperiled newborns seriously as something more than an abstract argument made by a tiny minority of misguided academics. Second, it will make a distinction between "healthy" and "imperiled" newborns and, in considering the arguments of Peter Singer, reply to the position that even healthy newborns are nonpersons. Third, in considering the arguments of Engelhardt, Fletcher, and Shelp, the chapter will reply to the position that *imperiled* newborns, specifically, are nonpersons.

Before proceeding, however, I want to highlight a very important point. In considering these arguments seriously the book in no way is

1. Michael R. Panicola, "Quality of Life and the Critically Ill Newborn: Life and Death Decision Making in the Neonatal Context" (Ph.D. diss., Saint Louis University, 2000), 112.

2. Engelhardt maintains that this is what a secular ethic must conclude. I am at pains in this chapter to show that this need not be the case.

3. For reasons that will become clear in chapter 4 (mostly having to do with having a controlled pool of resources), this book will mostly table the question of global distribution of resources — though such considerations could conceivably make its central argument even stronger.

endorsing the arguments against the moral status of newly born human infants. Indeed, precisely the opposite is intended: by taking on these arguments on their own terms, and showing them to be untenable, the book is arguing quite strongly for the personal dignity of even the most imperiled newborn human being. As will be shown in some detail, this dignity prohibits the direct, intentional killing of such neonates — but does not answer further questions about just distribution of resources.

## Some Historical Highlights

Issues of medical treatment of imperiled newborns are rooted clearly in practical, real-life situations that demand our attention. However, it might be less clear that theoretical questions regarding the moral status of such infants are equally as grounded. Later in this chapter several arguments will be bolstered by thought experiments that have theoretical but no practical application to our current technological reality. It is thus important — especially for a topic so rooted in real-life practical situations — that the central question of this chapter be given careful and unbiased consideration. If the claim that a newborn infant is not a person, in any context other than academic ethics, is just "too shocking to be taken seriously,"[4] then perhaps it is something like a "brute fact" that newborn infants are persons in the full moral sense of the word and the tiny minority of philosophers who hold this view should not even be given a hearing.[5]

But even if *today* this is the attitude toward the moral status of human infants (I will argue that this is not as clear as one might think), a quick look at ancient and more contemporary historical examples suggests that a very different attitude toward this question can be articulately defended. Direct infanticide has been a socially accepted practice, Singer points out, "from Tahiti to Greenland . . . and from the nomadic Australian aborigines to the sophisticated urban community of ancient Greece and mandarin China."[6] William Silverman claims that

4. Peter Singer, *Practical Ethics,* 2nd ed. (Cambridge and New York: Cambridge University Press, 1993), 172.

5. This is the reaction, in fact, of many neonatal physicians and nurses when presented with these kinds of arguments.

6. Singer, *Practical Ethics,* 172.

"Infanticide is the oldest method of human family planning" and that "child murder was common" in cultures preceding ours.[7] Lita Schwartz and Natalie Isser add that "neonaticide and infanticide have been practiced on every continent and by people on every level of cultural complexity, from hunters and gatherers to those in 'higher' civilizations, including our own ancestors and contemporaries. Rather than being the exception, it has been the rule."[8] Given the vast amount of historical material with which to work, this chapter will merely highlight examples from only two eras: ancient Greece and Rome, and the modern age.

## Imperiled Newborns in Ancient Greece and Rome

We begin with three cautions. First, in investigating every historical era one must consider the possibility (indeed, the likelihood) that there is a significant difference between theoretical values espoused in a text and actual cultural practice. Second, even if we end up concluding that practices are based on theoretical values, Earl Shelp asks us to consider that though these practices and values "might be viewed as regrettable, [they] could be *understood*, given the societal and cultural forces at work during any particular time and place." Indeed, it may be that they should not be seen as moral rogues, but instead as "people in crisis attempting more or less conscientiously to find their way."[9] Finally, we need to see a particular practice in its full historical context — not isolated in a vacuum. Perhaps the fact that Greece and Rome had many practices that actually respected human life would lead us to see their understanding of infanticide and exposure in a different light. These warnings will prove valuable not only in our brief historical exploration, but also in examining our own cultural situation with regard to these issues.

We know infants were exposed in the ancient Mediterranean, but

7. W. A. Silverman, "Mismatched Attitudes about Neonatal Death," *Hastings Center Report* 11, no. 6 (December 1981): 12-13.

8. Lita Linzer Schwartz and Natalie Isser, *Endangered Children: Neonaticide, Infanticide, Filicide*, Pacific Institute Series on Forensic Psychology (Boca Raton, Fla.: CRC Press, 2000), v.

9. Earl E. Shelp, *Born to Die? Deciding the Fate of Critically Ill Newborns* (New York: Free Press; London: Collier Macmillan, 1986), 163, emphasis added.

we need to know the *frequency* of the practice. If it was the exception rather than the rule,[10] perhaps we would take a different stance toward what the historical record shows. Consider a letter written by an ancient husband, Hilarion, to his pregnant wife Alis that dates from 1 B.C.E.: "Know that I am still in Alexandria. And do not worry if they all come back and I remain in Alexandria. I ask and beg you to take good care of our baby son, and as soon as I receive payment I shall send it up to you. If you are delivered of a child [before I come home], if it is a boy keep it, if a girl discard it. You have sent me word, 'Don't forget me.' How can I forget you? I beg you not to worry."[11] This is a remarkable passage. If he is being truthful in this letter, Hilarion is a man of deep feeling: along with the clear affection for his baby son, he loves his wife and attempts to ease her worry with this letter. However, this makes his matter-of-fact discussion about discarding his future daughter that much more jolting. How could someone with such deep affections be so cavalier about the exposure (and, presumably, death) of his daughter unless such a practice was tied to deeply held cultural beliefs about the moral status of such an infant? Indeed, a father in ancient Greece had a right to take some time to decide whether or not the newborn child would be welcomed into his family — a kind of second or "social" birth.

Though it seems clear that this era had a different understanding of the moral status of newborn infants than does our era, some complexities should be taken into consideration. For purposes of the topic of this chapter, and for the book's ultimate conclusion, we might make a distinction between the moral status of imperiled newborns who were often directly killed and those relatively healthy newborns who were often exposed. Though exposure was well known and socially accepted in ancient Greece and Rome, it was done for various reasons and in several ways — and these variables make the understanding of the moral status of these infants a complex matter indeed. In addition to exposure because a child was female, complex relationships with the gods also led to exposure — either in response to an omen of doom or as a protest to events considered gravely unjust.

10. Child "exposure" in the form of abandonment takes place in our culture as an exception rather than the rule. This, by itself, does not tell us much about our culture's attitude toward the moral status of infants.

11. Rodney Stark, *The Rise of Christianity: A Sociologist Reconsiders History* (Princeton: Princeton University Press, 1996), 98.

Though many affluent ancients exposed their children, by far the most common social reason for the practice was poverty. One more mouth to feed might all too easily mean taking food from family members who already suffered hunger.[12] Indeed, though many times exposure seems to have meant certain death, it appears some families had genuine hope that their children would be saved — leaving the infant at a street corner, near a public building like a temple, or even at spots just outside a city or village that were specifically designed for exposure. Such hope was not always misplaced. Though scholars disagree as to the rates of survival, it appears that at least some of these infants became foster children and less fortunate ones were picked up for later use as slaves or prostitutes.[13] The commonness of this kind of exposure may say less about the attitude of the parents or culture toward the moral status of such infants than about the social realities with regard to scarcity of resources — and the desperation that such scarcity would drive some families who clearly wanted to give their infant child a chance at life.[14]

These complexities notwithstanding, it seems clear that ancient Greeks and Romans did not consider newly born infants — whether healthy or imperiled — to have the same moral status as adults or even older children. The intellectual elite defended this view in theory and in law, and the data we have for the actual practice, though complex, seems to indicate that both direct killing and exposure of the newly born were common, and commonly accepted, events. One might be tempted to dismiss these historical considerations as relics of a time long past with virtually nothing to teach us. Slavery was also practiced in these cultures, and surely that historical consideration, all by itself, says nothing about the moral legitimacy of slavery for today. However, when these historical considerations are combined with an examination of our contemporary attitudes and practices (and cogent arguments), we have good reason to take this position seriously.

---

12. O. M. Bakke, *When Children Became People: The Birth of Childhood in Early Christianity* (Minneapolis: Augsburg Fortress, 2005), 30.

13. Bakke, *When Children Became People,* 31-32.

14. This distinction between moral status and actions (or nonactions) taken in light of scarcity of resources is an essential distinction for this book. Also important to note is the fact that ancient Christians were well known, and even made fun of, for rescuing such exposed infants. The fact that this is one of the identifying features of early Christianity will have implications for the conclusion of this book.

## Contemporary Attitudes and Practices

Even in today's world there is plenty of evidence that, upon reflection, perhaps we are not as sure about the moral status of infants as one might think. As John-Thor Dahlburg has pointed out, "in rural India, the centuries-old practice of female infanticide can still be considered a wise course of action."[15] According to Dahlburg, infants are killed in various ways: by feeding them dry, unhulled rice that punctures their windpipes; by making them swallow powdered fertilizer; by smothering them with a wet towel; or simply by allowing them to starve to death. Of 1,250 families studied by the Community Service Guild of Madras, 740 had only one female child and 249 admitted to having killed at least one female infant.[16] Nor is this problem limited to the 1990s. In March 2007 human rights groups launched a new campaign to combat infanticide in thirteen Indian districts. They report that "Killing baby girls soon after birth is widely practiced in poor southern districts of the state, with some areas reporting 15% death among female babies."[17] The Indian government has acknowledged the severity of the issue and has set up orphanages around the problem districts to raise abandoned baby girls in an attempt to halt the practice. The event that sparked the energy behind the initiative was the discovery of the remains of 400 female fetuses and newborns buried in a pit behind a hospital in the central Indian city of Bhopal. When asked if the scheme would encourage women to abandon their infant girls, Chowdhury said, "It doesn't matter. It is better than killing them."[18]

Lest one think modern examples of infanticide are limited to the developing world, it is worth looking at the so-called Groningen Proto-

15. John-Thor Dahlburg, "Where Killing Baby Girls Is 'No Big Sin,'" *Toronto Star,* February 28, 1994.

16. Malavika Karlekar, "The Girl Child in India: Does She Have Any Rights?" *Canadian Woman Studies* (March 1995).

17. Sampath Kumar, "India Rights Campaign for Infanticide Mothers," BBC News, July 17, 2003; http://news.bbc.co.uk/2/hi/south_asia/3071747.stm (accessed March 13, 2007).

18. "Indian Gov't to Raise Bandoned Girls," Associated Press, ABC News; http://abcnews.go.com/Health/wireStory?id=2884808&CMP=OTC-RSSFeeds0312 (accessed March 13, 2007).

col — named after a medical center in the Netherlands that created a public written proposal to permit physicians to actively end the lives of infants. Suitable candidates for infanticide fall into three categories:

1.  Infants with no chance of survival. This group consists of infants who will die soon after birth, despite optimal care with the most current methods available locally. These infants have severe underlying disease, such as lung and kidney hypoplasia.
2.  Infants with a very poor prognosis who are dependent on intensive care. These patients may survive after a period of intensive treatment, but expectations for their future condition are very grim. They have severe brain abnormalities or extensive organ damage caused by extreme hypoxemia. When these infants can survive beyond the period of intensive care, they have an extremely poor prognosis and a poor quality of life.
3.  Infants with a hopeless prognosis who experience what parents and medical experts deem to be unbearable suffering. Although it is difficult to define in the abstract, this group includes patients who are not dependent on intensive medical treatment but for whom a very poor quality of life, associated with sustained suffering, is predicted. For example, a child with the most serious form of spina bifida will have an extremely poor quality of life, even after many operations. This group also includes infants who have survived thanks to intensive care but for whom it becomes clear after intensive treatment has been completed that the quality of life will be very poor and for whom there is no hope of improvement.

Though infanticide[19] is still technically a crime in the Netherlands, the culture seems to support it in some circumstances — and the legal exceptions involve an appeal to desperate circumstances in which nothing else could be done. Despite national surveys suggesting that this

19. Those who are sympathetic to this kind of protocol might object to lumping it in with other procedures also described as "infanticide" in this section (killing infant girls based on gender, for instance). However, all that is meant by using this term here is the direct killing of an infant — not a moral equation with other kinds of practices. Indeed, the aim of this section is merely to present evidence that, perhaps, one should not be so quick to think that today's modern world simply accepts de facto that infants are full persons. Some evidence presented is stronger than other kinds.

kind of infanticide takes place fifteen to twenty times per year, no physicians have been prosecuted for it since the adoption of the protocol in 2002.[20] Nor is this is the only European country to have mixed attitudes toward the practice. The respected Royal College of Obstetricians and Gynecologists in England submitted a proposal to the Nuffield Council on Bioethics that urged them "to think more radically about non-resuscitation, withdrawal of treatment decisions, the best interests test and *active euthanasia* as they are ways of widening the management options available to the sickest of newborns."[21] Catherine Damme has shown that this kind of attitude has its roots in English common law, which treated infanticide as a separate offense from homicide in that it had a lesser punishment and established a very liberal insanity defense for mothers who committed infanticide.[22]

Even the United States has a problem with infanticide. According to Steven Pinker, "every year hundreds of women commit neonaticide," and in response, "Prosecutors sometimes don't prosecute; juries rarely convict; those found guilty almost never go to jail."[23] A CNN review of FBI statistics bears out the numbers. It appears that about five infants a week are killed in the United States — and interestingly, deaths of male infants are almost always higher in a given year than those of females.[24]

But perhaps more interesting than hard infanticide numbers are other indications of some American attitudes toward the newly born. During U.S. Senate debate over a bill that would have banned partial-birth abortion, the following exchange took place between Senators Santorum (R-PA) and Boxer (D-CA) on October 20, 1999.[25] A public ar-

20. E. Verhagen and P. J. Sauer, "The Groningen Protocol — Euthanasia in Severely Ill Newborns," *New England Journal of Medicine* 352, no. 10 (March 10, 2005): 959-62.

21. Sarah-Kate Templeton, "Doctors: Let Us Kill Disabled Babies," *Times Online*, November 5, 2006; http://www.timesonline.co.uk/tol/news/uk/article625477.ece (accessed April 4, 2007), emphasis added.

22. Catherine Damme, "Infanticide: The Worth of an Infant under Law," *Medical History* 22 (1978): 1-24.

23. Steven Pinker, "Why They Kill Their Newborns," *New York Times*, November 2, 1997. Many of these women are suffering from mental illness, but discussion of the complex issue of what our practices for prosecution of infanticide versus other kinds of homicide says about our understanding of the moral status of infants follows below.

24. "Nearly 5 Babies Killed Weekly, FBI Data Show," CNN, June 27, 1997; http://www.cnn.com/US/9706/27/killed.babies/index.html (accessed March 13, 2007).

25. The following is quoted directly from the *Congressional Record*, available at

gument in which a distinguished U.S. senator refuses to condemn infanticide on the floor of the U.S. Senate is powerful evidence about our current attitudes toward the moral status of newborn infants and bears full quotation. The issue being pressed by Senator Santorum is the moral status and treatment of a newborn infant and not the moral status of a fetus:

> MR. SANTORUM: But I would like to ask you this question. You agree, once the child is born, separated from the mother, that that child is protected by the Constitution and cannot be killed? Do you agree with that?
>
> MRS. BOXER: I would make this statement. That this Constitution as it currently is — some want to amend it to say life begins at conception. I think *when you bring your baby home* [emphasis added], when your baby is born — and there is no such thing as partial-birth — the baby belongs to your family and has the rights. But I am not willing to amend the Constitution to say that a fetus is a person, which I know you would. But we will get to that later. I know my colleague is engaging me in a colloquy on his time. I appreciate it. I will answer these questions.
>
> MR. SANTORUM: I ask the Senator from California, again, you believe — you said "once the baby comes home." Obviously, you don't mean they have to take the baby out of the hospital for it to be protected by the Constitution. Once the baby is separated from the mother, you would agree — completely separated from the mother — you would agree that baby is entitled to constitutional protection?
>
> MRS. BOXER: I will tell you why I don't want to engage in this. You had the same conversation with a colleague of mine, and I never saw such a twisting of his remarks.
>
> MR. SANTORUM: I say to the Senator from California, I am not twisting anything. I am simply asking a very straightforward question. There is no hidden question here. The question is —
>
> MRS. BOXER: I am answering the question I have been posed by the Senator, and the answer to the question is, I stand by Roe v.

Thomas.loc.gov (accessed April 4, 2007). Some nonrelevant or procedural text has been omitted.

Wade. I stand by it. I hope we have a chance to vote on it. It is very clear, Roe v. Wade. That is what I stand by; my friend doesn't.

MR. SANTORUM: Are you suggesting Roe v. Wade covered the issue of a baby in the process of being born?

MRS. BOXER: I am saying what Roe v. Wade says is, in the early stages of a pregnancy, a woman has the right to choose; in the later stages, the States have the right — yes — to come in and restrict. I support those restrictions, as long as two things happen: They respect the life of the mother and the health of the mother.

The discussion continues at some length about what would qualify as "birth" for Senator Boxer — and she simply claims over and over that "it is obvious" in response to Senator Santorum's pressing questions. Perhaps her difficulty in answering his questions is understood best in light of her using the striking phrase "when you bring your baby home" as describing birth in her original answer. Santorum simply dismisses this as too absurd to be believed and therefore a mistake, but this is too quick. Boxer here, though she retreats from the position, interestingly seems to have invoked the ancient Greco-Roman concept of *social* birth over and against mere biological birth. Why would someone want decisions about the infant born during a botched partial-birth abortion to be made by parents and physicians? At least one likely answer is that it is the parents and physicians themselves[26] who decide the moral status of newly born infants — they do not have the objective personal moral status of more mature human beings.

I have attempted to show that the claim that "all or some human infants are not full members of the personal moral community" deserves a place at the table in the debate over moral status. This claim has been explicitly held throughout history in cultures that varied widely in their practices and level of sophistication. And it seems to have not totally disappeared from view in our own culture — though its remnants are not as explicit as the attitudes and practices in older cultures. But because something was widely practiced in ancient times and still remains with us today is not by itself an argument for that practice — but it does clear the conceptual space needed for those who consider

26. This is also the position, as we will see later, of Engelhardt and Shelp when they invoke the concept of "social" personhood.

the abstract philosophical argument "too shocking to be taken seriously." The chapter now turns to specific philosophical arguments for the claim that either (1) all human infants are not full members of the moral community (Singer and Tooley) or (2) some imperiled human infants are not full members of the moral community (Engelhardt, Shelp, and Fletcher).[27]

## The Social Quality of Life Model
## and the Moral Status of Newborns

Recall that the major reason for invoking a strong version of the social quality of life model was that newly born human infants were not persons. Are there serious arguments that can defend the proposition that human infants are not persons and therefore deserve less medical resources than persons? A name consistently invoked in support of this version of the social quality of life model is Peter Singer, the Ira W. DeCamp Professor of Bioethics at Princeton University.[28] Richard Sparks, for instance, spends many pages discussing Singer's view that "if parents regret the child's birth and are truly burdened by the continued existence of a child," they have the "right to kill the infant in the name of their own social welfare."[29] This part of the chapter will take a detailed look at Singer's argument about the moral status of newborn infants.[30]

---

27. These are two different "families" of arguments considered in separate areas of the chapter.

28. Singer makes an argument for some strong version of the social quality of life model with regard to newborns several places, including the following: Helga Kuhse and Peter Singer, "Hard Choices: Ethical Questions Raised by the Birth of Handicapped Infants," in *Ethics on the Frontiers of Human Existence,* ed. Paul Badham (New York: Paragon House, 1992); Helga Kuhse and Peter Singer, *Should the Baby Live? The Problem of Handicapped Infants,* Studies in Bioethics (Oxford and New York: Oxford University Press, 1985), 228; Peter Singer, *Rethinking Life and Death: The Collapse of Our Traditional Ethics* (New York: St. Martin's Griffin, 1996), 115-31; Singer, *Practical Ethics,* 191-213. Most recently, he made a startlingly similar argument in "Why We Must Ration Health Care," *New York Times Magazine,* July 15, 2009; http://www.nytimes.com/2009/07/19/magazine/19healthcare-t.html (accessed August 10, 2009).

29. Richard C. Sparks, *To Treat or Not to Treat: Bioethics and the Handicapped Newborn* (New York: Paulist, 1988), 240.

30. Much of the argument about healthy newborn infants is borrowed from an ar-

Let us begin with Singer's principle of "equal consideration of interests," which entails that "we give equal weight in our moral deliberations to the like interests of all those affected by our actions."[31] Further principles are formed when this reasoning is applied to specific situations. Animals, Singer points out, have interests (say, in avoiding pain). Given this, Singer is able to morally condemn as "speciesist" those who "give greater weight to the interests of members of their own species when there is a clash between their interests and the interests of other species. Human speciesists do not accept that pain is as bad when it is felt by pigs or mice as when it is felt by humans."[32] Therefore, the *comparable* interests of nonhuman animals should factor equally into our moral considerations.[33] This does not necessarily mean, however, treating animals as morally equal to (all) humans. Singer admits that "the greater the degree of self-awareness and rationality and the broader the range of possible experiences, the more one would prefer the kind of life" — and thus "it would not necessarily be speciesist to rank the value of different lives in some hierarchical ordering."[34] Therefore, the *varied* interests of different beings allow us to rank their moral value in a hierarchy.

Things get messy, of course, when we start attempting to justify such a ranking. Singer spends quite a bit of time considering the moral status

---

gument I made about healthy fetuses: Charles Camosy, "Common Ground on Surgical Abortion? — Engaging Peter Singer on the Moral Status of Potential Persons," *Journal of Medicine and Philosophy* 33, no. 6 (December 2008).

31. Singer, *Practical Ethics,* 21.

32. Singer, *Practical Ethics,* 58.

33. Some might claim that such a principle is not at all neutral when it comes to infanticide — nor any other kind of killing of human organisms. Indeed, something like "speciesism" might be not only morally permissible, but perhaps morally *required.* Mary Midgley, (*Animals and Why They Matter* [Athens: University of Georgia Press, 1984]), for instance, argues that species preference is "an absolutely central element in human happiness" and "the root from which charity grows" (103). She suggests that it is "a necessary part of our social nature," and that, unlike racism, it is not "a product of culture" (105). But these claims are too strong, for even in Midgley's conclusion on this issue she claims only that "a developing social creature needs to be surrounded by beings *very similar to it*" (107, emphasis added). This is the admission that Singer would hammer — claiming that his position still stands. Mere species preference is not the relevant consideration, but rather social capacity and example.

34. Singer, *Practical Ethics,* 107.

of a person — that is, for him, "a rational and self-conscious being that is aware of itself as a distinct entity with a past and a future."[35] Singer is not clear whether he believes that persons have a right to life,[36] but he does believe that interest utilitarianism gives us good reasons for thinking that it is more serious to kill a person than a nonperson. Persons, because they can have plans for the future and are aware of themselves existing over time, would have their interest violated by being killed in ways that nonpersons would not. Because Singer is a *rule*-interest utilitarian — that is, he believes we should be "guided by a set of well-chosen intuitive principles" rather than attempting to "calculate the consequences of each significant moral choice"[37] — he can generalize about the moral value of persons. He says, "Killing a person who prefers to continue living is therefore wrong, other things being equal."[38] We now have a Singerian principle that is neutral with respect to infanticide:

> Other things being equal, it is wrong to kill a person (as opposed to a nonperson) because that person has an interest[39] in continuing to live.

The key question is whether or not an infant is a person with personal interests — that is, whether or not an infant (at least according to Singer's definition)[40] is "a rational and self-conscious being that is

---

35. Singer, *Practical Ethics*, III.

36. He claims that he is "not convinced" that the idea of a right to life "is a helpful or meaningful one" (Singer, *Practical Ethics*, 96). But because the idea is "popular," he considers whether there are grounds for attributing such a right to persons and not to nonpersons. He then launches into a discussion of Michael Tooley's argument — without coming to any conclusion on the matter. Later, however (172), he does speak of a "legal" right to life in the affirmative. His position is not clear.

37. Singer, *Practical Ethics*, 93.

38. Singer, *Practical Ethics*, 93.

39. I continue to use Singer's original word "interest" — rather than "preference" — for two reasons. First, when he makes the shift to "preference" (Singer, *Practical Ethics*, 94), he gives us no reason to accept it. Second, it seems clear that even if some person (say, a depressed junior high schooler) did not currently have the preference to continue to live, it would still be wrong to kill him because it was in his interest to continue living.

40. One might wonder why the chapter uses Singer's definition rather than arguing for one of its own. While it seems clear his definition of "person" needs some expansion and nuance, it is not incorrect — and, again, the point of this section is to defeat the argument on its own terms.

aware of itself as a distinct entity with a past and a future."[41] If an infant is not a person, there is no reason to accord its life any "greater value than the life of a nonhuman animal at a similar level of rationality, self-consciousness, awareness, capacity to feel, etc."[42] But an infant is not rational, not self-conscious, and not aware of itself as a distinct entity with a past and a future. He baldly states that "the grounds for not killing persons do not apply to newborn infants"[43] because infants, frankly, are not persons. They cannot reason and they certainly are not aware of themselves over time. Singer says there should be at least some circumstances in which a full legal right to life comes into force not at birth, but only a short time after birth — perhaps a month.[44] Here, then, is our key Singerian principle:

> Human newborn infants, because they are not persons, do not have a right to life and can be killed up until (at least) a month after birth.

## A Third Option?

Singer, quite neatly, paints an either/or situation for us. Either the human infant is a person with the actualized capacities Singer deems necessary for this kind of moral status, or the infant should be treated as having no greater value than a nonhuman animal at a similar level of capacity. Anything other than these two options is going to count as speciesism. But are these the only options open to us? A human infant may not qualify as an actualized person (as Singer defines the term), but it does not follow from this that the moral value of the infant needs to be located in her actualized capacities. A human newborn infant may not be any more rational or aware of herself in time than is a snail (as Singer points out), but there is an obvious distinction to be made between a snail and a newborn human infant — and that distinction lies in the *potentiality* of the infant. The snail can only develop as a

41. Singer, *Practical Ethics*, 151.
42. Singer, *Practical Ethics*, 151.
43. Singer, *Practical Ethics*, 171.
44. It is difficult to understand why Singer chooses this date, rather than one much later. Indeed, an infant at one month is nowhere near as mentally sophisticated as an adult chimpanzee or dolphin — a threshold one would think necessary for personhood even in Singer's system.

snail does — that is, morally speaking at least, not very much at all. The snail will never be able to love or feel love. The snail will never be able to have projects of its own. A snail will never self-consciously wonder about its place in the universe. The infant, under normal circumstances, will experience all these things. The infant will develop as a human organism does — as a rational creature with a sense of herself over time. That is, as a *person* as Singer defines it.

But because it is difficult to articulate, one might wonder just how the potential of the human infant and fetus is *morally relevant.* Indeed, even defenders of the personhood of human infants think appeals to potential are mistaken. Patrick Lee and Robert George, for instance, seem to argue that "we human beings have the special kind of value that makes us subjects of rights in virtue of *what* we are, not in virtue of some attribute that we acquire some time after we have come to be."[45] But what the human infant is, without some reference to future potential, is not more significant morally than a snail or a chicken — that is, without an appeal to future potential.[46] Any other kind of evaluation is wrongfully speciesist. Let us look at an often-cited example of someone who tries to take into account the future of an infant as it impacts her moral status.

## Don Marquis

Don Marquis is well known for his attempts to account for how the future potential of a human infant (and fetus) might be morally relevant. He starts with what he thinks is an unproblematic assumption: "it is wrong to kill *us.*" Why? "[T]he loss of one's life deprives one of all the experiences, activities, projects, and enjoyments that would otherwise have constituted one's future." These things are "either valuable for their own sakes or means to something else that is valuable for its own sake."[47] In

---

45. Andrew I. Cohen and Christopher Heath Wellman, *Contemporary Debates in Applied Ethics,* Contemporary Debates in Philosophy, vol. 3 (Malden, Mass.: Blackwell, 2005), 17.

46. This book makes the argument that the "kind of thing" an infant is cannot be separated from the "future potential" she has for morally relevant attributes. Much more on this to come.

47. Don Marquis, "Why Abortion Is Immoral," *Journal of Philosophy* 86 (1989): 189.

addition, there are most probably goods in one's future that, while not currently valued, will "come to be valued by me as I grow older and as my values and capacities change." Therefore, what makes killing "*any* adult human being"[48] seriously wrong is the "loss of his or her future."[49] Marquis uses this basic insight to draw several conclusions:

1. It is false that it is wrong to kill beings only that are biologically human. Alien species on other planets, for instance, could have a future like ours. It might be seriously wrong to kill them.
2. There is at least the possibility that some nonhuman animals have a future like ours and it might be seriously wrong to kill them.
3. Active euthanasia of some adult human beings who do not have a future like ours might not be wrong.
4. It is *prima facie* seriously wrong to kill children and infants because they have a future like ours.
5. It is *prima facie* seriously wrong to kill fetuses because they have a future like ours.[50]

Marquis articulates the potential of the human infant and fetus as her capacity to have "a future like ours" and locates not only *her* moral status in this potential, but *everyone's* moral status in this potential. It is an intuitively convincing argument — one that has generated quite a bit of response literature — but not one, I think, without important problems.

Indeed, one might wonder, as Peter McInerney does, if conclusion 5 above is as obvious as Marquis thinks it is. McInerney argues that because of "the complexity of the biological and psychological connections between earlier and later stages of one person," "the claim that a fetus has a personal future in the way that a normal adult human has a personal future" is invalidated.[51] He claims that though "there is some biological continuity between them so that there is a sense in which the

48. One might ask here what Marquis means by this phrase. Does he mean literally *any* adult human being? What about an adult human in a permanently comatose state? In fact, he does not mean to include such a being — and the fact that he is not more specific creates a problem for his project.

49. Marquis, "Why Abortion Is Immoral," 190.

50. Marquis, "Why Abortion Is Immoral," 190-92.

51. Peter K. McInerney, "Does a Fetus Already have a Future-Like-Ours?" *Journal of Philosophy* 87, no. 5 (1990): 264-68, here 265.

later person stages 'are the future' of the fetus, the fetus is so little connected to the later personal life that it cannot be deprived of that personal life."[52] He cites Derek Parfit's theory that psychological relations
between temporal "selves" constitute personal identity (if it even makes
sense to call it this) through time.[53] He notes that there are three
"widely considered" kinds of relations: "memory, continuity of character, and intention-to-action."[54] Because personal identity consists in
these kinds of psychological relations, and because there is no psychological relation between a fetus and a "future" in which the same biological animal has such relations, it is simply false to say that a fetus
has "a future like ours." Also, it follows from this argument that not
only are human fetuses without moral status, but human infants are
without it as well. Indeed, many infants are not connected via memory
to their future, nor do they have "continuity of character" with their
future biological self, nor can they form intentions to act on the future.
By any standard used to argue that a human fetus does not have a *personal* future like ours, a human infant would fail to have the same future using the same standard.[55]

But the human fetus and infant are not the only ones in danger of
losing moral status given this paradigm. Consider a human being in a
light coma that the doctors have determined, when she wakes, will have
severe amnesia — that is, she will not remember who she is. Like the fetus or infant, she is not currently psychologically connected in the ways
that McInerney deems necessary to talk about her having a personal
future like ours. Surely we cannot deny her the moral status of a person. If the McInerney test is the one to be met, we end up with absurd
ethical conclusions.

<hr />

52. McInerney, "Does a Fetus?" 267.

53. Obviously, it is beyond the scope of the chapter to engage this theory adequately, but I have argued elsewhere that Parfit's theory is problematic in the moral conclusions one is forced to draw from its application.

54. McInerney, "Does a Fetus?" 265.

55. Perhaps dreading this implication, McInerney notes that the "possibilities that
are available to a person or even to a young infant are not now available to the fetus"
(McInerney, "Does a Fetus?" 267). But it is hard to see what such possibilities would be,
and why they would be relevant to the psychological connections he puts forth. Again, if
memory, character, and intention are the relevant relations, a newborn infant is just as
lacking in these qualities as is a fetus.

But while Marquis moves the debate in the proper direction — toward the moral value of the potential future of the infant and away from discussion about actualized capacities — he needs to be pushed further. A key question is who *counts* as "us" in his assumed dictum: *it is wrong to kill us.* Apparently because it would be "difficult" and "controversial," Marquis admits that he has no "additional account of just what it is about my future or the futures of other adult human beings which makes it wrong to kill us."[56] But can he get away with not coming down on this issue? He sees this question as related only to specific questions regarding whether certain animals have a future like ours, but it is not clear why this is the case. Suppose that *just what it is* that is morally valuable about my future (that which makes it wrong to kill me as opposed to another being without a future like mine) is that I will be rational and aware of myself in time — Singer's definition of personhood. This would allow for not only the abortion and infanticide of many thousands of mentally disabled human beings, but also the killing of such human beings as older children or adults. Did former President Reagan, as victim of mental illness such that his future would never be rational or aware of himself in time, have a future like ours? If the answer is no, then we end up denying moral status to Reagan and all those like him in mental capacity — but if the answer is yes, then what nonhuman animals *would* qualify for full moral status? On what basis would one deny dogs, chickens, or even snails full moral status? No, Marquis is on to something here, but he needs to say more about what precisely it is about our futures that makes denying them morally problematic.[57]

It seems that one may accept Singer's definition of an actualized person — a being that is rational and aware of itself in time — but argue that this is not the only way to talk about the kind of moral status that Singer wants to reserve only to actualized persons. It is the central thesis of this chapter that beings that are *potential persons* — to use Singer's categories, those beings that are potentially rational and aware of themselves in time — have the same moral status as beings with actualized rationality and self-awareness in time. This is what accounts not

56. Marquis, "Why Abortion Is Immoral," 191.
57. Perhaps, as we will soon see, it has something to do with the kind of being something is — the potential inherent to a being's nature. This would reflect the insight of Lee and George cited above.

only for our moral intuitions regarding infants, but also for many other adult human beings. The enraged, the extremely intoxicated, the asleep, the insane, and the temporarily comatose are all human beings that fail to meet Singer's actualized criteria for personhood — but virtually no one denies these beings moral status. This charge argues that the reason is because of their potentiality for rationality and/or awareness of themselves in time at some point in the future.[58] And it is precisely for this reason that moral status should also be extended to human infants and fetuses.

## Objections to the Argument from Potential

As Massimo Reichlin notes in his "Argument from Potential: A Reappraisal," the argument from potential (AFP) "does not have a good press in today's . . . debate."[59] This is certainly not overstatement. Even Don Marquis, who makes an argument very similar to the AFP, calls its basic inference "invalid."[60] Others are harsher. Those who object to the AFP seem to make two general kinds of arguments, the "no interest" (NI) argument and the "problems with probability" (PP) argument:

1. If only those with the proper interests can have moral status, then a potential person cannot have moral status because it has none of the relevant interests. Indeed, many kinds of things might be "potential persons" but do not have the interests proper to persons and therefore cannot have moral status. (NI)
2. If every potential person has moral status, this leads us into problematic questions about the relationship between probability and possibility. Is any being that has a probability of becoming a person greater than zero a "potential person"? If the answer is yes, this may lead us to absurd conclusions about what counts as having

58. Certainly many proponents of theories like Singer's interest view disagree and try to locate rationality, etc., in such beings in light of their having had rational interests (and the like) in the past. But the chapter will show that such arguments are fundamentally mistaken.

59. Massimo Reichlin, "The Argument from Potential: A Reappraisal," *Bioethics* 11, no. 1 (January 1997): 1.

60. Marquis, "Why Abortion Is Immoral," 192.

moral status. If the answer is no, then we have a problem with deciding at what level of probability of becoming a person is granted "potential personhood" — and therefore moral — status. (PP)

Peter Singer, Ronald Dworkin, and Michael Tooley all make different versions of the NI argument. Singer claims that "the fact that the embryo has a certain potential does not mean that we can really harm it, in the sense that we can harm a being who has wants and desires or can suffer."[61] Indeed, if "it is claimed that destroying an embryo does it harm because of the loss of its potential, why should we not say the same about an egg and sperm?"[62] Would we consider a laboratory technician blameworthy for rinsing spare ova and sperm down a drain and causing the loss of potential personhood?[63] A sperm-egg pair, considered jointly, is surely a potential person — but it cannot have interests and therefore cannot have moral status. In the same way, a newborn infant is a potential person, but because it cannot have interests it also cannot have moral status.

Dworkin's version of the NI argument is very similar to Singer's. He claims that "it is very hard to make sense of the idea that an early fetus has interests of its own" — for, in order to have interests, it is not enough that it might "grow or develop into a human being."[64] He asks us to consider an assemblage of body parts on the laboratory table of Dr. Frankenstein. Suppose that just as the good doctor was about to throw the lever that would give the assemblage life, an individual (apparently appalled by the experiment) smashes Dr. Frankenstein's machine. We would not, of course, consider the individual blameworthy for harming the assemblage of body parts. But, Dworkin argues, if the assemblage is a potential person, then the AFP insists that it *has* been harmed. But this is absurd because the assemblage clearly has no interests of its own and cannot be harmed.

61. Singer, *Rethinking Life and Death,* 97.
62. Singer, *Rethinking Life and Death,* 99.
63. Depending on what part of Singer one is reading, he speaks about either potential life, potential human, or potential person as if they were interchangeable. I use "personhood" here because I assume this is what he must respond to in order to answer AFP as presented here.
64. Ronald Dworkin, *Life's Dominion: An Argument about Abortion, Euthanasia, and Individual Freedom* (New York: Knopf, 1993), 16.

Michael Tooley, another supporter of infanticide, gives perhaps the most interesting version of the NI argument.[65] Tooley asks us to imagine that in the future it will be possible to inject kittens with a chemical that will endow them with capabilities consistent with human personhood. These injected kittens would then have moral status because they would be rational and aware of themselves in time. But would we think a stray kitten was seriously wronged if someone, upon finding it, refused to inject it and instead handed it over to animal control to be painlessly euthanized? The kitten does not have the morally relevant interests to be wronged as a person, but given the injection technology, it appears that it is a potential person. Given the AFP, it then also appears that the kitten should have the same moral status as a person — and would be wronged by the person who did not inject it. But this is absurd.

## Response to the "No Interest" Objections

What can one say in response to these versions of NI? An obvious first move is to table this whole discussion for the moment (it will be addressed below) and point out again that a friend of NI must have answers to questions about our moral intuitions regarding the enraged, the extremely intoxicated, the asleep, the insane, and the temporarily comatose. It looks as if, because NI requires that a being currently have the relevant personal interests to have moral status, regardless of its potential to have them in the future, the above examples are beings that a friend of NI must claim are without moral status.

Bonnie Steinbock claims that in each example above the being in question has had the relevant interests "in the past." This past is relevant because it forms "the basis for saying that the comatose person wants not to be killed while unconscious." Indeed, killing adult humans is different from killing human fetuses or infants "because they have a life they (ordinarily) value and which they would prefer not to lose."[66] Appar-

---

65. Michael Tooley, *Abortion and Infanticide* (Oxford: Clarendon; New York: Oxford University Press, 1983), 191-93.

66. Bonnie Steinbock, "Why Most Abortions Are Not Wrong," *Advances in Bioethics* 5 (1999): 245-67.

ently, a comatose adult human continues to have such an interest, while an infant or fetus lacks just such an interest. Daniel Dombrowski and Robert Deltete argue in a similar way. They point out that "a car mechanic who is not currently fixing cars" can "still legitimately be called a car mechanic."[67] In the same way, a person who currently does not have interests that are personal can still legitimately be called a person.

What follows are simple forms of the argument being put forth:

1. Joe is not now acting as a car mechanic.
2. Joe has acted as a car mechanic in the past.
3. Therefore, Joe can still be considered a car mechanic.

1. Joe is not now acting as a person.
2. Joe has acted as a person in the past.
3. Therefore, Joe can still be considered a person.

OK, but what about the following argument?

1. Charlie is not now acting as the third baseman for St. Joseph's High School.
2. Charlie has acted as the third baseman for St. Joseph's High School in the past.
3. Therefore, Charlie can still be considered the third baseman for St. Joseph's High School.

Of course, this conclusion is absurd. I am now many years removed from having been the third baseman at SJHS and I have *no potential in the future* to ever be so again. My past is wholly irrelevant to the question of whether or not it is legitimate to call me the third baseman at SJHS, and what *is* relevant is my future potential. The same can be said of Joe. If Joe never again fixes a car, and is now not currently fixing cars, in what sense *is* it legitimate to still call him a car mechanic?

A thought experiment might help clarify this point. If Michael Tooley can speak of injecting cats with a drug that can turn them into persons, perhaps I can be forgiven for speaking of a *Star Trek* "replicator

67. Daniel A. Dombrowski and Robert Deltete, *A Brief, Liberal, Catholic Defense of Abortion* (Champaign: University of Illinois Press, 2007), 78.

machine." Let us take Joe, a human being in a temporary, light, and induced coma, and put him into the replicator and throw the switch. Now we have Joe 1 and, his identical "clone," Joe 2 — both comatose, and both exactly the same in every other respect. Both, when we bring them out of their comas, will have certain important interests that would have been thwarted by killing them. Let's say that before replication, Joe 1 (according to both friend and foe of NI) wanted to get married and have children, continue his education, and look after his sick mother. Presumably, he still has these interests after replication. But what about Joe 2? It looks as if those who support the NI must argue that Joe 2 does not have moral status and may be killed without violating any of these important interests. After all, Joe 2 — like a human infant — has not had personal interests in his past that can be said to be operative while he is currently comatose. If it is the past that matters, and not the future, then Joe 2 may be killed without wronging him. But someone arguing that killing Joe 2 (who is in every way other than his past indistinguishable from Joe 1) is wrong would want to argue that Joe 2's coma is temporary and that his future potential for personal interests grants him the moral status of a person. After all, when he wakes, he will articulate the exact same interests of Joe 1. If this intuition is correct, then it is the *future* that matters — not the past. And it is for this reason that the infant should be considered to have moral status.

But perhaps one should want to go in the *other* direction. Perhaps one might simply admit that every being that does not have personal interests cannot have moral status. Therefore, even if counterintuitive to our moral sensibilities about the moral status of infants and the temporarily comatose, one needs to bite the bullet and take the road down which the argument leads. But this need not be the case. Both Singer and Steinbock (and they are not alone) fluctuate back and forth between talking about interests and preferences[68] as if they were the same thing. Clearly they are not. What might be in one's best interests is often

---

68. We have already noted where Singer did this. Steinbock does this when she flat-out admits that "Our interests also include what is *in* our interest, whether or not we are interested in [that is, *prefer*] it" (Bonnie Steinbock, "Respect for Human Embryos," in *Cloning and the Future of Human Embryo Research*, ed. Paul Lauritzen [Oxford and New York: Oxford University Press], 25), and then proceeds, as already noted, to claim that what makes killing an adult human being wrong is that it (ordinarily) values its life and prefers not to lose it.

*not* what one prefers. Many children would *prefer* not to go to school, but a parent who allows such a child to skip school nevertheless violates the child's *interest* — because going to school is in the child's best interest. This, then, is the way out for one who wishes to ground moral status in interests. The enraged, the extremely intoxicated, the asleep, the insane, the temporarily comatose, the human fetus, and the human infant can be described as having certain states of affairs being in their best interests — but, again, it is all based on their *future* potential.[69]

## The "Problems with Potential" Objection

But a wholly different kind of argument against the AFP, remember, is the following:

> If every potential person has moral status, then this leads us into problematic questions about the relationship between probability and possibility. Is any being that has a probability of becoming a person greater than zero a "potential person"? If the answer is yes, this may lead us to absurd conclusions about what counts as having moral status. If the answer is no, then we have a problem with deciding at what level of probability of becoming a person is granted "potential personhood" — and therefore moral — status. (PP)

R. Alta Charo makes an interesting version of the PP in her *Every Cell Is Sacred: Logical Consequences of the Argument from Potential in the Age of Cloning.*[70] Charo points out that with the advent of human cloning, every single cell is now a potential person — even though the probability of a particular cell becoming a person is extremely small. If we are not to get just as worried about killing our skin cells as we are about killing infants

69. Here is another example. Suppose a twelve-year-old boy prefers to die because he has just broken up with his junior high girlfriend — and he overdoses on pain pills, which put him in a light coma. Now suppose someone kills him. His being killed violates none of the backward-looking preferences that Singer and Steinbock claim are necessary. But it seems obvious that his killer did violate an *interest* of his — and the only way to make sense of this claim is with reference to *future*-looking considerations.

70. In Paul Lauritzen, *Cloning and the Future,* 291. Her argument is most persuasive as a defense of destruction of human fetuses outside of a mother's womb, but it is worth bringing up in this context as well.

or fetuses, we need to deal with the problem of probability. Why does one level of potential personhood "count" morally but another level does not? Roy Perrett points out that some have tried to figure out a probability marker for moral status. He cites Roman Catholic ethicist John Noonan's 80 percent mark — which Noonan believes is the probability a fetus will become a person — as an example. This number appears to contrast with the probability that a body cell will become a person to a degree that makes it acceptable that the fetus should count as a potential person and the body cell should not. But, Perrett argues, this marker will not work for fetuses before week six gestation because "more recent research has altered our best estimate of the real probabilities"[71] and before week six a fetus has less than an 80 percent probability of becoming a person.[72] Consider each of the following:

1. A body cell with an infinitesimally small probability of becoming a person.
2. A fetus at sixteen weeks gestation with an 80 percent probability of becoming a person.
3. A fetus at five weeks gestation with a 55 percent chance of becoming a person.
4. A fetus at ten weeks gestation that a doctor, due to complications in the pregnancy, gives a 10 percent chance of becoming a person.

On what basis, those who make Perrett's claim ask, can one claim that (2), (3), and (4) above should count as having moral status but (1) should not?[73] Perrett also asks an important question about implications of the AFP and potentiality in other areas of life: "Why should the 80% probability of becoming an X give something the rights of an actual X? Even if it is now true that Prince Charles has an 80% probability of becoming king, this does not presently give him the rights of an actual king. Why should it be any different for fetuses?"[74]

71. Roy W. Perrett, "Taking Life and the Argument from Potentiality," *Midwest Studies in Philosophy* 24 (2000): 186-98, here 189.
72. Indeed, if the research Perrett cites is correct, before week six (but postimplantation) the probability is anywhere from 46 percent to 60 percent.
73. Or, alternatively, that (2) and (3) should count as having moral status but (1) and (4) should not.
74. Perrett, "Taking Life," 189.

These are important and intuitively plausible arguments. Can a friend of the AFP respond? One thing that surely needs to be highlighted here (in *both* the NI and the PP) is what appears to be a conflation of the concept of potentiality with probability and/or mere possibility. Reichlin has pointed out that "a correct understanding of the embryo's potentiality shows that by progressively acquiring new capacities — including the capacity to perform rational operations — the human individual develops and perfects the human nature it already possesses."[75] Reichlin then moves to an Aristotelian distinction between *active* and *passive* potency. A tree, in its passive potency, is a *possible* table — however, this does not mean in any sense that a tree is already a table. Active potencies, by contrast, "are those inherent to the very nature of the being, whose principle of actualization is the very nature of that being."[76] No external agent is necessary, and the potentiality is "the capacity to express and actualize inherent potentialities towards which the being in question has a natural tendency — i.e., a tendency which is dependent on its very nature."[77] A fertilized acorn, then, is a potential oak tree — but because this potential *is part of its very nature,* this means that the acorn is already, in some sense, an oak tree.

This argument, in addition to answering the PP (which we will get to presently), provides another reason to reject some versions of the NI argument. With regard to a move like Singer's to consider a "sperm and egg jointly," Perrett notes that "a gamete is not even a potential embryo, but rather depends essentially on external causes. The human sperm does not just need a proper place wherein to develop its inherent potentialities, but needs an external event which is going to change radically its identity and potentialities."[78] Thus, if by "potential person" we mean something with *active* potency for personhood and not merely passive potency, the moral difference between a fetus and a sperm or ovum becomes clear. Like the comatose adult, a fetus has an active potency in its potential personhood, but a gamete has mere passive potency for personhood — making it a *possible* person, but not a potential person. The same can be said of Dworkin's assemblage of body

75. Reichlin, "The Argument from Potential," 12.
76. Reichlin, "The Argument from Potential," 17.
77. Reichlin, "The Argument from Potential," 16.
78. Perrett, "Taking Life," 13.

parts. While it is certainly a possible person, because it would take "an external event which is going to change radically its identity and potentialities" for it to actually become a person, it is therefore not a potential person in the morally relevant sense. One can also see how this move works with Tooley's kitten thought experiment. Even if the "personhood injection" existed, kittens would have only passive potency for personhood. That is, they are *possible* persons in the same way a tree is a possible table and a sperm is a possible person. Each would need an outside event, separate from its becoming something inherent to its nature, to become the thing in question. The event of a kitten being injected is akin to the ovum being fertilized or the tree being cut down and made into a table — in the process of changing it has lost its original nature and become something else.

We can also see now how this responds to Charo's and Perrett's probability questions. Sure, a body cell may (given cloning) have a certain very low probability of becoming a person — but this is the wrong question to ask in determining whether or not the cell is a *potential* person. We need to find out whether a body cell has an active or passive potency for personhood. It seems clear that, because a body cell will not of its own nature turn into a person, it would rely on an *external outside event*[79] to do so — thus making it a *possible* person and not a potential person. Perrett's Prince Charles example meets the same fate. To use Reichlin's language, Prince Charles's becoming king "is in fact dependent on several external causes, such as social conventions and regulations, and in no way implies the kind of necessity shown by a natural development."[80] Prince Charles's 80 percent probability of becoming king has nothing to do with his nature — and this is why it makes sense to not treat him as if he were the actual king. But at sixteen weeks gestation Prince Charles had an 80 percent probability of becoming a person, and because this was due to his *nature* it *did* make sense to treat him with the moral status of a person.

Thus the arguments against the AFP considered here appear to have

79. Charo's important point is that if one considered the zygote as a subject of stem cell research — outside the womb — it appears that it is only a possible person and not a potential person. She suggests this makes it reasonable to do research on human embryos even given the AFP. I leave this claim unanswered for two reasons. First, it gets into complicated questions about the moral issues in creating IVF embryos that are beyond the scope of the book. Second, again, the focus of this argument is on newborn infants.

80. Reichlin, "The Argument from Potential," 6.

been answered. Indeed, as Lee and George nicely summarize it, an entity having moral status (as opposed to having a right to perform a specific action in a given situation) follows from "an entity's being the *type of thing* (or substantial entity) it is. And so, just as one's right to life does not come and go with one's location or situation, so it does not accrue to someone in virtue of an acquired (i.e. accidental) property, capacity, skill, or disposition. Rather, this right belongs to the human being at all times that he or she exists, not just during certain stages of his or her existence, or in certain circumstances, or in virtue of additional accidental features."[81] Of course, much depends on accepting the distinction that Aristotle and Reichlin make between active and passive potency (or between essential and accidental properties) — as well as the concept of "nature" inherent in the distinction. But we've seen that Singer does accept the concept of a human nature, and the distinction between a tree becoming a table (passive potency) and a fertilized acorn becoming an oak tree (active potency) is convincing and would require significant work to rebut. In addition, we have seen that it is difficult to understand the moral status of those who have temporarily lost actualized personal capacities without reliance on this concept of "nature" used in the AFP.

But what if the opponent of the AFP asks: What is to be done with human beings who appear *not* to be potential persons? We have already mentioned examples of these: those with advanced Alzheimer's disease, the severely autistic, the permanently comatose, etc. If we accept the AFP, it appears that such individuals cannot have moral status — for, because they can never again be rational or aware of themselves in time, they are neither persons nor potential persons. If we accept as a brute fact that the above human beings do in fact have moral status, then it appears that the AFP fails.

Singer, or any other ethicist that locates moral status in (either potential or actual) personal interests, is going to be stuck with this problem. If such ethicists want to defend some kind of moral worth in the above human beings, they appear to be forced to make a Steinbock-like move[82] of distinguishing between moral *status* and moral *value*. The former would be applied to persons and the latter to other beings and

81. Cohen and Wellman, *Contemporary Debates,* 17.

82. As described in Maura Ryan, "Creating Embryos for Research: On Weighing the Symbolic Costs," in *Cloning and the Future of Human Embryo Research,* 53.

things that have a different kind of value. Perhaps those with advanced Alzheimer's disease, the severely autistic, and the permanently comatose are "potent symbols of human life" — and for that reason have some significant moral value and, while lacking full moral status, nevertheless deserve some moral respect.[83] The weakness of this move, of course, is that without moral status the lives of such human beings could easily be trumped by the interests of actual or potential persons — and thus allow for ending their lives to serve those interests. Perhaps the responsible thing to do is to kill those with Alzheimer's and autism to conserve resources to support the interests of actual or potential persons. But I think most of us would find this morally repugnant. Maybe we ought to take our cue from Singer at this point, bite our lips, and just accept our repugnant conclusion. After all, if there truly is (as he would have us believe)[84] a "Copernican revolution" going on in ethics, why should we expect that the conclusions we come to will be comfortable? Such conclusions would apply not only to mature human beings with these disabilities but also to the subject of this book: similarly imperiled newborns. The vast majority of those who hold the social quality of life model for treatment of imperiled newborns do so precisely because they believe they do not have full moral status.

## The Moral Status of *Imperiled* Newborns

To this point, the focus of the chapter has been on the moral status of *healthy* newborn infants; to be sure, if a healthy newborn infant is not a person, then it certainly follows that an imperiled newborn is not a person and thus would require far less moral consideration (and, therefore, treatment) than would actual persons. But let us now consider the possibility that while *healthy* newborns are persons, certain *imperiled* newborns are not. After all, these are the kinds of babies in the NICU. For purposes of this chapter imperiled newborns will fall into four different categories — each with a specific case[85] to exemplify and reference it.

83. Ryan, "Creating Embryos for Research," 55.
84. Singer, *Rethinking Life and Death*, 188 and 256.
85. I owe many of the ideas for this section to Steve Leuthner, M.D., M.A. (bioethics) — a neonatologist at Children's Hospitals of Wisconsin and head of its ethics committee.

**Case #1, "Annie"** — Very Severe Mental Disability, Terminal

Annie was born with anencephaly — a nonrepairable lesion of the central nervous system based on a defect of neural tube development. While there are reports of maintaining these children on life support for a few years, only rarely does the infant not get an infection from the typical open skull. Annie has some brainstem activity such as suck and swallow reflexes and may actually feed. She has no cerebral cortex, and if there are neurons present they are totally unorganized and not part of a functional organ. She is having seizures, however, which has led to some palliative medication need. Her prognosis is terminal within the first days to weeks of life.

**Case #2, "James"** — Severe Mental Disability, Not Terminal

James was born with a severe case of hypoxic-ischemic encephalopathy (HIE) — brain damage as a result of asphyxia. He is virtually nonresponsive, and even on his best days as a child James won't even be able to recognize his mother. Yet, in some HIE children parents can perceive some pleasure/pain experiences. For example, they may say the baby groans when near the end of gastric-tube feeding, or coos some sort of way when they brush the baby's hair. What level of consciousness the child has is difficult to prove. Typically these children are cortically blind, often deaf, not capable of any true speech/language/communication other than guttural sounds. Typically they are close but don't reach the current definitions of persistent vegetative state. James's prognosis is that the HIE will endure, but he is not terminal.

**Case #3, "Patrick"** — Moderate Mental Disability, Not Terminal

Patrick was born with "Fragile X" Syndrome — a mutation of the FMR1 gene on the X chromosome. He is sweet and loving and exhibits a strong desire for social interaction, but is severely learning-disabled with an IQ likely in the mid-30s. Patrick will probably be able to communicate, but will need to do so using pictures or sign language. He will also need a tremendous amount of help with basic things like sleeping, eating, dressing, using the restroom, and hygiene. There is no cure for Fragile X, but it is not a terminal condition.

**Case #4, "Christopher"** — No Mental Disability, Not Terminal

Christopher was born with gastroschisis and has lost all his intestines from a volvulus (twisting of the intestines until they infarct). There is no reason to suspect any major injury to the brain and therefore to suspect any neurological impairments. The only option seems to be to maintain him on total parenteral nutrition (IV) in hopes of him growing big enough to get a bowel transplant before there is the toxicity of liver failure. Typically there will be liver failure, so if he gets big enough, he will need both a liver and a bowel transplant. The success of getting to the age to do that is low, as is the success of the transplant itself. And even if the transplant is successful, Christopher (and his parents) will have a life of chronic medical and financial burdens.

How should friends of the social quality of life model evaluate the cases of these imperiled newborns? We know Singer would consider them all nonpersons simply for being infants. Here we examine the views of three other ethicists who support "strong" views of the model: physician-philosopher H. Tristram Engelhardt Jr., philosopher Earl Shelp, and theologian Joseph Fletcher. While these three ethicists admit that healthy newborns are persons (or, for all practical purposes, should be treated as if they were persons),[86] they also believe that certain imperiled newborns should be treated as something less than full persons. Thus, they hold the strong view for some imperiled newborns for the same reason that Singer holds it for all newborns.

## H. Tristram Engelhardt Jr.

In some ways, Engelhardt is the most like Peter Singer of these three thinkers. However, this requires a major caveat: Engelhardt is a Christian and believes he must be committed to the proposition that infanticide is morally wrong (though not necessarily murder) as part of his Christian identity, but he tries to argue from the point of view of a secular ethic to show its limitations. Indeed, he claims: "When one examines the contrast between traditional Judeo-Christian understandings of the status of embryos, fetuses, infants and reproduction, the difference between what can be established in general secular morality and in

---

86. Engelhardt and Shelp speak of the "social" (as opposed to objective) personhood of healthy newborns, however. More on this distinction to come.

traditional Judeo-Christian appreciations is most stark. It is impossible to make out the evil not only of abortion but infanticide."[87] Under such a secular ethics, Engelhardt argues, only rational, self-conscious, and morally autonomous beings are persons in an objective, strict sense.[88] This means that some human beings — especially the very young or disabled — do not count as persons in this sense. But they may qualify as persons in a *social* sense. What this means substantively is not clear, but at a very basic level it refers to entities (usually humans, though based on this definition there is no reason to limit it in this way) on whom a certain level of moral status is conferred "justified in terms of utilitarian and consequentialist reasons." Such justifications will be "somewhat different" depending on the situation, but Engelhardt offers three criteria by which we might consider an entity a person in the social sense:

1. It would support important virtues such as sympathy and care for human life — especially when it is fragile and defenseless.
2. It would offer protection against the uncertainties of when exactly humans become persons — as well as those who have various levels of incompetence.
3. It would secure the practice of child rearing through which humans become persons in the strict sense.[89]

For Engelhardt, healthy newborns will generally qualify as persons in the social sense, but for *imperiled* newborns a set of considerations will often show that they would not qualify. He explains that "there are secular moral grounds for not imposing undue financial and psychological burdens on those who are persons in the strict sense" as long as they are not violating the interests of innocent persons and judging "that a defective newborn should either be allowed painlessly to die (or even be aided in dying painlessly!) do not offend against [this constraint]."[90] That is, such defective newborns do not count as persons in either the strict *or* the social sense.

87. H. Tristram Engelhardt, *The Foundations of Bioethics* (New York: Oxford University Press, 1986), 277.

88. Engelhardt, *The Foundations of Bioethics*, 137.

89. Engelhardt, *The Foundations of Bioethics*, 147-48.

90. Engelhardt, *The Foundations of Bioethics*, 148.

Though evaluating the benefits against the burdens in these situations is often tricky and much of the time done on a case-by-case basis, Engelhardt does come up with some general principles for attempting to think about evaluating in the abstract. The strength of a case to treat an imperiled newborn on the basis of its being a person in the social sense can be determined, roughly, by taking the chance of success of the treatment multiplied by the probable quality and length of life of the child and dividing by the costs of the treatment:

$$\frac{\text{Chance of Treatment Success} \times \text{Probable Quality of Life} \times \text{Length of Life}}{\text{Cost}}$$

Armed with this algorithm and his underlying philosophy, we can see how Engelhardt would evaluate the cases.

Annie certainly would not qualify as a person in the social sense for Engelhardt. The chance of treatment success is zero. This is enough for a final judgment to be made, but the probable quality of life is also zero and the length of life is near zero. Cost may be relatively low, especially considering the length of life, but with a numerator of zero this really is inconsequential in Engelhardt's scheme.

Treatment of James has a good chance of success — that is, simply on a biological level of keeping him physically alive. However, James's prospects for quality of life are not much different than those of a fairly simple nonhuman animal — perhaps a chicken or a mouse. And though HIE cases usually involve a significantly shorter life span, it is not necessarily dramatic enough to affect our calculation here. The costs of treating James throughout his life, however, are quite dramatic given his limitations — not the least of which will be for a full-time caregiver. But how do the overall numbers break down for James? Engelhardt is not very clear about how to "score" certain aspects of his algorithm — but one might be justified in giving him a zero for quality of life if one needs a quality of life that has *some* future prospect for rationality, autonomy, and self-consciousness. However, even if the quality of life is not zero, it is a very small number, and when pitted against the very high costs associated with keeping him alive, it seems that Engelhardt's view would still prohibit James from attaining social personhood.

Patrick is much like James from the standpoint of treatment and life span. However, he has significantly better prospects for quality of life. Rather than simply "cooing" and having very basic pleasure/pain experience, Patrick is a social creature who can interact with other persons — and even communicate using nonverbal means. Though somewhat less costly than James's — especially long term — Patrick's care is still very expensive. Though his case is more difficult to call than James's, he is not a good prospect for Engelhardt's social personhood. Certain nonhuman animals, who are not considered persons,[91] appear to have a similar quality of life — dolphins and primates, for instance, have similar social relationships and communication skills. Couple that with the very significant cost of treatment and, though it is a much more difficult call than James or Annie, Patrick appears to fall short of the mark.

Though Christopher does not have a terminal disease in the strict sense,[92] he certainly has other problems. The chance of the treatment's success is very low — and though there is a prospect for a life that is not overly short, that quality of life will likely be lowered by the medical burdens from future treatment. Also, cost is, again, a significant factor. There seem to be enough low numbers for Christopher here that, like Patrick, his case is not a slam dunk, but he does not seem like a good candidate for social personhood.

However, were a family to accept an infant[93] and "assign her the role of child within an established set of practices, perhaps by accepting social support in various fashion for the child's care and development,"[94] things could change. Then even the above imperiled newborns might qualify for personhood in the social sense. However, the focus of

91. As Singer and others have pointed out, rather than claiming that Patrick is not a person, perhaps we should expand our notion of person and instead grant dolphins, primates, and perhaps some other nonhuman animals full moral status.

92. What counts as a terminal disease is certainly open to question. While anencephaly is clear-cut, this case is not — Christopher need not necessarily die from the disease, but social factors often play a role in making this determination. If treatment for a disease is not available because of one's social situation, or is simply too burdensome, then one could argue that such a disease is terminal as well.

93. Once again we are reminded of the ancient Greek practice of family acceptance of an infant for moral status to be conferred.

94. Engelhardt, *The Foundations of Bioethics*, 149.

this chapter is on the moral status of infants in the NICU — generally a stage of life before such bonding and assigning take place.[95] Given that situation, it must be admitted that the four examples above are poor cases for social personhood in the Engelhardt model.

## Earl Shelp

Shelp argues, much like Engelhardt, that certain newborn infants are to be considered persons in the social sense rather than in a strict objective sense. An infant qualifies for this status insofar as she can make demands on her parents and community to protect and preserve her life. Such a duty obtains proportionally to an infant's ability to maintain "personal independence" — which is indisputably a "primary end toward which parental activity should be directed."[96] The kinds of characteristics that indicate personal independence, for Shelp, include the newborn's capacity "to relate, communicate, ambulate, and perform tasks of basic hygiene, feeding, and dressing."[97] If a newborn infant has "an incapacity to attain a minimum level of independence," then it is appropriate to take account of the needs of other persons — especially married persons and more mature siblings — and give them priority over the neonate. Shelp sees it as "intuitively unfair or unjust to sacrifice the opportunity of a healthy child in order to sustain the existence of a severely defective or impaired brother or sister."[98] The choice in these kinds of situations "is not between two competing equals," and thus it is not unfair to prefer "the interests of the healthy over the interests of the imperiled."[99] Indeed, Shelp argues that "par-

95. Of course, one could certainly argue that one need not wait until after birth (or even birth itself) for such bonding and assigning to take place. Perhaps a mother and/or father would have accepted the child *in utero*, at which point social personhood may have been conferred. However, if this is possible, it confuses us about what social personhood is substantively. Is it simply whatever a parent decides it is? Or can a parent simply decide when to make the social connections that would bring it into effect? If yes, then social personhood means whatever we want it to mean — and Engelhardt's point that this confusion is a product of a "content-less" secular ethics is laid bare.

96. Shelp, *Born to Die?* 46.

97. Shelp, *Born to Die?* 48.

98. Shelp, *Born to Die?* 137-38.

99. Shelp, *Born to Die?* 76.

ents of severely diseased or defective newborns may reasonably choose not to authorize life-prolonging interventions" when "it is reasonably believed that the infant's condition is such that the capacities sufficient for a minimal independence or personhood" cannot be attained.[100]

Unlike Engelhardt, Shelp does not come up with a calculus for determining social personhood, but rather puts imperiled newborns into three diagnostic categories:[101]

1. Newborns with medical conditions that cannot be effectively treated. No prospects for attaining a minimum level of independence and thus social personhood.
2. Newborns with medical conditions that could be effectively treated and could produce a normal or near-normal quality of life. High probability of attaining independence and thus social personhood.
3. The third category, unlike the first two, presents significant complexity and open-endedness. In these cases therapeutic interventions are available, but the projected quality of life is very poor.[102] In such cases, the family should be given much latitude in weighing this kind of imperiled newborn's interests against the interests of the family. In general, the interests of persons in the family should take precedence over those infants with a limited capacity to sustain future independence.

How would Shelp evaluate the four cases above? Shelp would agree with Engelhardt that the case of Annie is not a close call — but rather than using any kind of calculus, he would simply mention that the capacity for a minimal level of personal independence is not present and therefore neither is social personhood. She falls into the first category above.

James, an infant who needs to be fed through a gastric tube and whose level of consciousness is difficult to prove, doesn't appear to

100. Shelp, *Born to Die?* 203.
101. Shelp, *Born to Die?* 126-27.
102. By "poor" Shelp apparently means non- or minimally autonomous, non- or minimally relational, and (interestingly) "a level of life purchased at an incommensurate cost" (Shelp, *Born to Die?* 127). Spelling out a version of this last point will be the focus of chapter 4 of this book.

meet Shelp's criteria for minimal independence and certainly cannot "ambulate and perform tasks of basic hygiene, feeding, and dressing." However, because James is not terminal, he falls into the third category above where a parent would have to weigh James's interests against the interests of those persons who are affected (parents, children, etc.). However, it is clear that James's personhood — if he has it — is merely a function of whatever his parents decide about the relative weight of the interests involved. He is not a person in any objective sense of the word.

Patrick, though he may have a dramatically different quality of life than James, nevertheless fails to have the kind of personal independence that Shelp requires for social personhood. He has a strong desire for social interaction — but will also need a tremendous amount of help with basic things like sleeping, eating, dressing, using the restroom, and hygiene, which preclude a minimum level of independence. Like James, Patrick's interests will need to be balanced against the personal interests of his family.

With Christopher, however, Engelhardt and Shelp may part company — for though his treatment is expensive, burdensome, and likely not to be successful, Christopher has good prospects for independence if he can beat the odds. The case is complicated, though, by the extreme cost and medical burden that would be a part of Christopher's treatment. It depends on whether or not the medical burdens of Christopher's life are commensurate with the cost of treatment. Again, for Shelp, this would be something parents or other family members would need to weigh for themselves.[103]

## Joseph Fletcher

Like the other two thinkers, Fletcher connects his "strong" view of the social quality of life model to the moral status of newborns. Unlike them, he rejects the "social" personhood approach and instead agonizes over what certain *objective* indicators of personhood might be:

---

103. This book will be at pains to argue that it is not merely a matter for the family, but rather the *broader community* if we are paying for the infant's current and/or future health care. The question of whether or not it is commensurate cannot be answered without an appeal to the burden of the *community* — not just the individual or family.

minimal intelligence, self-awareness, self-control, a sense of time, a sense of futurity, a sense of past, relational ability, concern for others, curiosity, and neocortial function all played major roles in his exploration.[104] However, he eventually comes to the conclusion that the most important quality is that which is "required for the presence of the others" — namely, neocortial function.

> Neocortial function is the key to humanness, the essential trait, the human *sine qua non*. The point is that without the synthesizing function of the cerebral cortex (without thought or mind), whether before it is present or with its end, the person is nonexistent no matter how much the individual's brain stem and mid-brain may continue to provide feelings and regulate autonomic physical functions. To be truly Homo sapiens we must be sapient, however minimally. Only this trait or capability is necessary to all of the other traits which go into the fullness of humanness. Therefore this indicator, neocortial function, is the first-order requirement and the key to the definition of a human being.[105]

Fletcher, then, has the least required to "count" a person — and also makes no distinction between a person in the objective sense and one in the social sense.

How would the individuals in our cases fare under Fletcher's standard? They are much easier to determine given his simple criteria. Annie does not have a neocortex and so clearly does not count as a person. James has a neocortex, but it is damaged to the point where its function does not permit personal "indicators" like self-awareness and relationality — so he also does not count as a person. Patrick's problem is the mutation of a gene — and not brain damage to the neocortex — and thus he would qualify. Christopher's problems have nothing whatever to do with the neocortex, and thus he would also qualify. Fletcher's view is, by far, the most friendly to imperiled newborns in terms of their moral status.

---

104. Joseph Francis Fletcher, "Four Indicators of Humanhood: The Enquiry Matures," *Hastings Center Report* 4, no. 6 (1974): 4-7.

105. Fletcher, "Four Indicators of Humanhood," 5-6.

## Critical Evaluation

How can we respond to the three approaches to the moral status of these imperiled newborns? The first aspect that must be called into question is shared by Engelhardt and Shelp: the distinction between objectively inherent personhood and socially bestowed personhood. In what sense is what they mean by "socially bestowed personhood" anything like personhood at all? Objectively inherent personhood, though more controversial when specifics are invoked, is, uncontroversially, something that refers to the dignity of the *entity bearing the name*. Though it certainly obligates others to respect that dignity by taking certain kinds of actions and refraining from others, the focus of the concept is *the dignity of the subject*. Socially bestowed personhood, by contrast, at least in the way Engelhardt and Shelp use the concept,[106] has nothing to do with anything objectively inherent to the infant — but rather with either (1) the social utility of the parent and/or community treating the infant in certain ways or (2) virtually whatever a parent decides about the balance of interests within a family. In this sense, such infants are persons in a very similar way to how a corporation is viewed as a "person" under American law — not because of any objectively inherent dignity the corporation has, but because of the social utility that comes from treating a corporation in certain ways. Given this purely instrumental way of using the term, virtually anything that, if we treated it in certain respectful ways that resembled how we treated persons, gave us a net benefit of utility could be considered a person in the social sense. But this is an evacuation of meaning from the phrase to the point where another term should be used — for most people mean something dramatically and categorically different from this when using the term in its objectively inherent sense.

Furthermore, we need not use such a term. Both Engelhardt and Shelp connect social personhood directly to the duties of parents and others in the community toward their infant children. But we can easily speak about the duties of, say, "owners to their animals" without calling animals persons. If Engelhardt and Shelp mean something very

---

106. One could use a concept of "socially bestowed personhood" in a way that coheres with a corresponding objective personhood. This, however, is not what is going on with Engelhardt and Shelp.

different from objective personhood, then a different term should be used. In using "socially bestowed personhood" they do not mean personal moral status — indeed, they are much like Singer in that they do not think these infants have any objectively inherent personal moral status at all. Given this, their arguments ultimately fall in the same way Singer's fall. They miss the implication that an infant's potential, rightly described, has for her moral status.

Given this limitation of the social quality of life model, perhaps Shelp could be rescued by taking his "capacity for a minimum level of independence" and turning it into an *objectively inherent* criterion. This could be a rival candidate to Singer's objective "rationality and self-awareness" criteria used above. Unfortunately, it does little better. Connecting independence to personhood almost completely misses the empirical reality of human personhood. Shelp notes that "no man is an island," but this is surely radical understatement. No human being has his identity as a person from anything other than (mostly dependent) relationships with others: with one's family, friends, God, communities and institutions, and so on.[107] A defining characteristic of human personhood is not independence, but interrelated *inter*dependence. Especially in today's globalized reality where small changes can send shockwaves through virtually all the economies of the world, it is precisely our radical *lack* of independence that has been laid bare for all to see.[108] Strongly connecting personhood with independence misses the anthropological mark.

But what of Fletcher? He certainly gets it right in searching for an objectively inherent indicator of personhood, but is his choice of "neocortial function" a good one? It would seem that it is not — for lots of other animals have neocortial function who do not have self-awareness and relationality (among other indicators), which, he says, constitute mature human persons. Rather, it is the *potential* for these other "mature" personal indicators that he really values as morally sig-

107. We will see this argument made in some detail in chapters 2 and 3.

108. In addition, for those that believe in a triune God whose very nature is one of interdependence of three persons in one being, we should hardly be surprised that human persons, made in the image of this triune God, mirror that kind of relationality in our personal natures. For a nice explication of this connection, see Catherine Mowry LaCugna, *God for Us: The Trinity and Christian Life* (San Francisco: HarperSanFrancisco, 1991), 243-92.

nificant. However, he mistakenly thinks that neocortial function is the "that without which" such traits could never come to be. Human organisms have several such organs of which the mature indicators will never come to be, if the organs do not develop (or develop properly). If he wants something more "basic," Fletcher should have gone back to an even more primitive indicator than development of the neocortex: that of the somatically integrated organism. It is this entity, and not a cerebral cortex in the abstract, that has the kind of potential for the indicators that Fletcher truly thinks are morally significant.

But now we have returned to the argument of the previous section that refuted Singer's position. Recall Reichlin pointing out that a human organism's "potentiality shows that by progressively acquiring new capacities — including the capacity to perform rational operations — the human individual develops and perfects the human nature it already possesses."[109] This potentiality is "the capacity to express and actualize inherent potentialities towards which the being in question has a natural tendency — i.e., a tendency which is dependent on its very nature." And it is "inherent to the very nature of the being, whose principle of actualization is the very nature of that being."[110] Existence of a human organism, then, with natural potential for personhood, is the true *sine qua non* indicator for personhood. Indeed, it is simply not the case, as Fletcher argues, that one need be "sapient" to be considered *Homo sapiens* — rather, one simply needs to be an organism with a natural potential for personhood.

But if the previous evaluations of the four cases fail, how should they be evaluated? How does the concept of personal moral status as being indicated by an organism with a natural potential for personhood "work" in these practical situations? The evaluation will not take long. All four are examples of human organisms with a natural potential for personhood — and thus count as persons in the moral sense. Christopher surely counts for he has no serious impairment that would call into question his being a human organism. Indeed, if the medical treatment he receives is successful, he will develop his natural potential into explicitly personal capacities. Patrick also has no impairment that would cause us to doubt his status as an organism. Indeed, if

---

109. Reichlin, "The Argument from Potential," 12.
110. Reichlin, "The Argument from Potential," 16-17.

genetic therapy existed that could cure him of his disease, he would also develop his natural potential for explicitly personal capacities.[111] James is also undoubtedly a human organism despite his brain damage. For if we were to find a way to repair the damage — say, by inserting cultured stem cells from neural tissue into the damaged areas — he would also express natural potential he had all along as a human organism. Finally, though this is surely counterintuitive for some people, Annie is also a human organism with the natural potential for personhood. Though she is profoundly disabled, she still has all the potential that every other member of her species has — but that potential has been frustrated by unfortunate circumstances.[112] No, all four examples are of human persons — and therefore these approaches to the "strong" social quality of life model seem to fail.

111. Some might argue here that Patrick's potential for gaining personal capacities is actually a fiction. No such treatment exists and thus the potential is zero. However, this is the same mistaken notion of potential that Charo uses earlier. It is mathematical potential (or "probability") rather than potential of kind or nature. Such mathematical potential can be influenced by a host of factors that have no moral relevance — many of them social. Consider that an infant born with bone cancer may have a mathematical probability of becoming a person of zero given her social situation (say, she is born in the remote areas of a developing country with no technology to treat such a disease), but that means nothing for her *actual* moral status — in light of her natural potential for personhood. Indeed, such potential would be realized if she lived in a different social situation. The same is true of Patrick (and also James and Annie) — if their social situations were different, their natural potential would be realized and thus they should be considered persons. However, this does not mean that all persons (including the four in the cases above) should therefore be treated. Though it is important to establish the full moral status of newborn infants from the start, the question whether or not these persons should receive full medical treatment is a very different one.

112. For some, this conclusion about anencephaly might be too quick. Might there be important differences between, say, James's brain damage and Annie's lack of a neocortex? Perhaps, but one would then have to make an argument as to what precisely this difference might be. We are currently just as unable to "fix" the brain of either James or Annie — and both are clearly human organisms with a natural potential for personhood. (Again, this is an argument about *moral status* only — and the arguments about *treatment* for James and Annie would be quite different. One might say that while both are persons, treatment of James would be mandatory but, for Annie, it might be burdensome.)

## One Final Challenge: The Argument of John Lizza

But the idea that those who are radically disabled (like an anencephalic infant) are persons in the same sense as more mature humans with a functioning rational and self-aware capacity is, for some, so counter-intuitive as to seem absurd. John Lizza makes a powerful argument that underpins such a reaction.[113] He argues that the best theoretical framework for thinking about persons is one that considers them "constituted by but not identical to human organisms."[114] The idea that any human organism at all has the natural potential for personal qualities and therefore counts as a person "invokes the most remote and promiscuous sense of *potentiality*."[115] For Lizza, a "more sensible, realistic concept of potentiality would support the claims that the life histories of persons and human organisms can diverge and that a person can die even though the organism that constituted it may remain alive."[116]

Indeed, Lizza claims that we can think of many human organisms that have this "remote and promiscuous" sense of potentiality that virtually no one would want to admit are persons. Though some of the examples he uses ask us to suspend disbelief and do a thought experiment, they are certainly worthy of serious consideration. What about a human body that has experienced whole brain death but has been artificially sustained? Or how about a human body that has been decapitated, but through futuristic technology is also artificially sustained? What about dead organisms? After all, sometimes dead butterflies are carefully mounted in museums and advertised as "members of their re-

---

113. John P. Lizza, *Persons, Humanity, and the Definition of Death* (Baltimore: Johns Hopkins University Press, 2006), 212.

114. Lizza, *Persons,* 96.

115. Lizza, *Persons,* 105.

116. Lizza, *Persons,* 100. Though Lizza is invoked here as a foil for the argument from potential as applied to imperiled newborns, one might wonder how he would talk about indicators of personhood in his own view. He talks about the need for a "biological substrate" (108) being necessary for personhood — rather than simply species membership. However, this kind of argument has already been answered above in the response to Fletcher. Lots of species that aren't persons have the same biological substrate as humans at the infancy stage — but it is only the natural potential for personal capacities that has moral weight. And this is contained in the organism herself — not in an adult cerebral cortex or embryonic primitive streak.

spective species" — why shouldn't we think that human cadavers, even after rigor mortis has set in, are also members of our species who, through some futuristic technology, might be brought back to life?[117]

If one thinks that any of the above examples counts as a person, Lizza suggests, then something has gone seriously wrong. For then "there is no rational basis for determining when such a radical power or potency for intellect and will is present in a thing" — the possibility that *anything* could become rational or self-aware cannot be ruled out, given advancing states of technology. In addition, he asks, "why should we think that the power remains" in any of these beings "as opposed to thinking that the power has left the body at this point?"[118] None of these beings will regain rational capacity "in the natural course of events." In fact, artificially sustaining or reanimating these bodies "falls outside the natural or normal course of events." Indeed, "if we were to do this, we intervene in the life history of the organism in such a radical way that we create new kinds of beings, and we should recognize that the human being or 'person' has died."[119]

Though Lizza isn't necessarily making an argument about imperiled newborns,[120] his views play directly into — and provide a direct challenge to — the central argument of this chapter. For, if the argument from potential means that entities like decapitated human bodies and even *dead* human bodies count as persons in the full moral sense, then it must be admitted that the view has been reduced to the absurd. Perhaps Annie, and even James and Patrick, rather than being human organisms who have stopped "constituting" a person,[121] are human organisms who have *never* constituted a person. If so, positions that support the social quality of life model based on the arguments of Engelhardt, Shelp, and Fletcher would need to be affirmed.

But there is an important response to Lizza's move here. He himself gives a clue to what it might be when he says that "if we were to do this, we intervene in the life history of the organism in such a radical way that we create new kinds of beings, and we should recognize that

117. Lizza, *Persons,* 105-6.

118. Lizza, *Persons,* 106.

119. Lizza, *Persons,* 107.

120. Though it is interesting that in arguing for his "biological substrate" model he discusses how anencephalic babies would not qualify. Lizza, *Persons,* 108.

121. Lizza, *Persons,* 100.

the human being or 'person' has died." We recall the discussion about Dr. Frankenstein's assemblage of body parts, Tooley's personhood-injected kittens, and Charo's cloned body cell. In each case there was first one "kind" of being — some disorganized tissue, a nonrational organism, and a cell that was part of another organism — that underwent a *nature-changing event*. The disorganized tissue was changed into that of an artificially animated creature with a personal nature. The kitten had its nature changed into an organism with a personal nature — indeed, it would no longer belong to the species of cat to which it had belonged previously. The body cell had its nature changed into an organism with a personal nature as well — instead of being part of another organism, she is now *her own* organism.

Lizza asks us to think about a "reverse" nature-changing event — the death of a person. Aren't (totally) brain-dead or decapitated bodies that are artificially sustained, or a body in which rigor mortis has set in, examples of beings that are the result of a nature-changing event? They once constituted beings with a personal nature, but after a nature-changing event (the death of the person) they no longer have such a nature. And if they were, through futuristic technology, to constitute persons again sometime in the future, that would also be a nature-changing event. It is not as if they would be persons the entire time.

This seems to be exactly right — and fits with the argument from natural potential leveled against Singer earlier. Recall that the claim was that all those with a natural potential for personhood should count as persons — and that newborns (healthy and imperiled) have this potential based on their biological membership as organisms in the species *Homo sapiens*. While it is true that a certain level (perhaps very high) of artificial sustenance is sometimes necessary to keep a human organism alive (artificial heart, ventilator, etc.), it does not follow that *any* human body that has certain physiological functions (like blood circulation and breathing) artificially sustained counts as an organism that is a member of *Homo sapiens*. Indeed, it is simply the case that though beings that are obviously dead (like the butterfly) may be corpses that "belong to a certain species," they are certainly not *organisms*. One could argue quite convincingly that the decapitated and whole-brain-dead corpses, artificially sustained, are in fact no longer organisms. Their animation is no longer simply aided or assisted by artificial means; that artificial means is now *itself responsible* for the animation. There is no longer an organism animating herself (with or without artificial assistance).

Admittedly, as with many binaries (such as alive/dead), there are gray areas that are difficult to distinguish. When does artificially assisted animation by the organism herself end and animation by the artificial means itself begin? Offering a definitive answer to this in the abstract surely gets us into complex questions of philosophy of biology,[122] but it seems one could discuss the cases of Annie, James, and Patrick without having to get too far into those questions. If we were to use artificial means to cure the disease of each of these beings, would they undergo a nature-changing event? Would they go from human organisms without a natural potential for personhood to human organisms with such natural potential? It seems clear that the answer to this question must be no. Whatever therapy used to treat their maladies (stem cell injections, gene therapy, etc.) would not create or instill a new natural potential. Instead, it would repair the injuries that are inhibiting the inherent natural potential from becoming actualized. If cured of their disease, these human organisms would be able to fully animate all aspects of their nature — including their personal capacities. Though Lizza's argument is a powerful one, and should be taken very seriously when we are thinking about brain-dead human bodies that are artificially sustained, it should not cause us to retract the view that all human newborn infants (both healthy and imperiled) are persons in light of their natural potential.

## Conclusion

History, and even a self-critical look at our present Western culture, shows us that the strong version of the social quality of life model — the view that at least some newborn infants are not full persons in the moral sense — far from being "too shocking to be taken seriously," must be carefully considered. It cannot be dismissed out of hand as ab-

---

122. For a good discussion of the nitty-gritty details of his complex question, see Kevin Elliott, "An Ironic Reductio for a Pro-Life Argument: Hurlbut's Proposal for Stem Cell Research," *Bioethics* 21, no. 2 (2007): 98-113.

surd or obviously wrong. That said, if the central argument of this chapter is correct, then the justifications for such a proposition (with respect to either all infants or simply certain imperiled ones) have failed to pass muster. This failure is important for two reasons. The first and most obvious reason is that this strong version of the social quality of life model relies on a faulty moral anthropology — a faulty notion of personal dignity and moral status. Second, because all newly born infants have the dignity and worth of persons, the good of their lives cannot be directly acted against in infanticide. We will see more about this line-drawing in the next chapter.

However, the direct killing of infanticide needs to be distinguished from the very different questions surrounding whether or not to medically treat an imperiled newborn. For some, the fact that all infants are full persons in the moral sense becomes a "conversation stopper" when the issue of factoring in social considerations in treatment decisions is raised. A discussion of this point of view is the focus of chapter 2.

# Arguments against the
# Social Quality of Life Model

*If we can say of adults (who can and do have obligations) that it is reasonable to expect that they will want a certain good for others and contribute to these goods if there is discernible risk, discomfort, or inconvenience, it is not precisely because they are adults that we conclude this, but because they are social human beings.*

Richard McCormick[1]

For a substantial number of those who share the conclusion of the previous chapter, discussion about whether social factors should be considered in determining whether or not to treat an imperiled newborn should now be over. Once we have established the full moral personhood of the infant, we know all we need to know. Personal dignity certainly cannot be reduced to social utility or to the amount of resources one is "worth." Such calculations, at a very basic level, deny the dignity of the individual human person that was established in chapter 1. Such radical individual dignity cannot and should not be subsumed within a broad social calculus about what is best for the community.

Indeed, isn't it the case that the modern discipline of bioethics has arisen largely as a response to, and safeguard against, precisely this kind of impoverished reasoning? Haven't foundational documents like the

---

1. Richard A. McCormick, "Experimentation in Children: Sharing in Sociality," *Hastings Center Report* 6 (December 1976): 41-46, here 42.

Nuremburg Code (a response to the medical abuses of the Nazis, who elevated the good of the community over the dignity of certain undesirable individuals), the National Research Act of the United States (a response to the medical abuses of the federal government, which ignored the dignity of certain African American individuals in the Tuskegee syphilis studies), and the World Medical Association's Declaration of Helsinki all claimed, in one way or another, that the autonomy and dignity of the individual cannot be reduced to the good of the community? This kind of reasoning seems to be especially important for physicians whose relationship with their patients is the foundation of medicine. Indeed, the World Medical Association's Declaration of Geneva makes claims that a physician must "always act in the patient's best interest when providing medical care" and to have "the health of my patient" as her first priority. This "patient's best interest" standard has been interpreted by modern clinical organizations like the American Association of Pediatrics Committee on Bioethics Policy to mean that the only benefits and burdens to be considered by the physicians are those that belong to the child (patient) alone.[2] This standard has been interpreted still further by the President's Commission for the Study of Ethical Problems in Medicine and Biomedical and Behavioral Research to "exclude consideration of the negative effects of an impaired child's life on other persons, including parents, siblings and society."[3]

These powerful and persuasive positions in today's modern bioethical culture fly in the face of the central argument of this book — which directly connects the benefit or burden of a treatment to just distribution of resources toward the common good — and thus deserve careful consideration. This chapter will attempt to address them in the following way. First, the chapter will consider arguments that rule out social considerations (at both theoretical and practical levels of inquiry) when deciding whether or not to treat an imperiled newborn. This view will be answered by a review of the Christian tradition on the distinction between ordinary and extraordinary means, which, from the point of view of this book, is clear and convincing about at least the

2. M. R. Mercurio, "Parental Authority and the Patient's Best Interest," *Journal of Perinatology* 26 (August 2006): 454.

3. President's Commission for the Study of Ethical Problems in Medicine and Biomedical and Behavioral Research, *Deciding to Forego Life-Sustaining Treatment* (Washington, D.C.: U.S. Government Printing Office, 1983), 218.

theoretical importance of social factors — due in no small part to the essentially social nature of the individual. Next, the view that while social factors in treatment decisions have some theoretical value they nevertheless should not be considered in practice — as articulated by Richard McCormick and John Paris — will be examined. These authors will be answered with both an internal critique of their positions and an attempt to show that their concerns about abuse are outweighed by claims of distributive justice. Next, the chapter will consider the argument by John Arras that this type of reasoning is de facto wrongful discrimination against disabled persons. The response to this argument will be that one need not factor in disability (as defined by Arras) into the calculation at all — but rather only cost (broadly speaking) as it relates to distributive justice. The chapter will then consider the arguments of Michael Panicola and Edmund Pellegrino that the very foundations of medicine are threatened by the social quality of life model in that it forces physicians to consider something other than their patient's best interests. The response to this argument will be that the concept of a patient's "best interest" — especially when viewed within a lens of Catholic social teaching and a relational anthropology — must be broadly construed to include the interest of affected others. The chapter will conclude with a recounting of the Ramsey/McCormick debate over whether nonautonomous children should be held to the same moral standard in this area as are adults — finding McCormick to have the stronger argument.

## Ruling Out Social Factors on Theoretical and Practical Levels: Paul Ramsey

James Walter attempted to summarize various ethicists' positions on the central question of this chapter: "For most of the authors under review, any inclusion of quality-of-life considerations into the decision to forego life-preserving treatment must be directly related to a *patient's* best interest. . . . Though the criteria of 'best interests' can be somewhat ambiguous, most would define it by reference to an assessment of the proportion of benefits and burdens of the treatment. If the burdens of the treatment *considered in itself* clearly outweigh any benefits *to the patient,* then it is morally permissible never to start or to terminate the treatment in question."[4] Though clearly many (perhaps even most) bioethicists strictly focus on the patient apart from social factors at both theoretical and practical levels of inquiry, this chapter will focus on a paradigmatic example in its analysis: the "medical indications" model of Protestant ethicist Paul Ramsey.

One of the important points Ramsey emphasizes is that most of the issues raised in medical ethics are not "special" or "unique" — they are manifestations of ethical issues that arise in personal relations more generally. Ramsey brings important Protestant Christian emphases to this discussion, one of which is a Christian understanding, revealed in Scripture, of *covenant*. He notes that "at crucial points in the analysis of medical ethics, I shall not be embarrassed to use as an interpretive principle the biblical norm of *fidelity to covenant*, with the meaning it gives to *righteousness* between man and man."[5] He agrees with Karl Barth that "covenant-fidelity is the inner meaning and purpose of our creation as human beings, while the whole of creation is the external basis and condition of the possibility of covenant. This means that the conscious acceptance of covenant responsibilities is the inner means of even the 'natural' or systematic relations or roles we enter by choice, while this fabric provides the external framework for human fulfillment in explicit covenants among men. The practice of medicine is one such covenant."[6] Questions like those being considered in this book involve "the principal task of medical ethics," which is "to reconcile the welfare of the individual with the welfare of mankind."[7] Crucial to this discussion is one's "view of man" because from this follows "the moral claims upon us in the crucial medical situations and human relations in which some decisions must be made about how to show respect for, protect, preserve and honor the life of fellow man."[8] Ramsey describes the principles that follow from these moral claims as "canons of loyalty" that exist between human beings generally, but also in specific instances within medicine.

4. James J. Walter, "Termination of Medical Treatment: The Setting of Moral Limits from Infancy to Old Age," *Religious Studies Review* 16 (October 1990): 303.

5. Paul Ramsey, *The Patient as Person: Explorations in Medical Ethics*, Lyman Beecher Lectures at Yale University (New Haven: Yale University Press, 1970), xii.

6. Ramsey, *The Patient as Person*, xii.

7. Ramsey, *The Patient as Person*, xiii.

8. Ramsey, *The Patient as Person*, xii.

One canon of loyalty for which Ramsey argues implies that "it is never right to turn against the good of human life. In the case of one's own life, public policy could go so far as to place that in the area of liberties. But to allow private individuals to turn against the good of another's life would be to promote injustice."[9] This position has at its heart the central idea that "an individual human life is absolutely unique, inviolable, irreplaceable, non-interchangeable, not substitutable, and not meldable with other lives."[10] This dignity is something we find in an embodied existence and is an essential, constitutive part of that dignity; therefore, when we choose against this embodied good (as when we deny potentially lifesaving treatments of another), we violate this dignity in an unacceptable, unjust way. To be sure, life-sustaining treatment can be withdrawn or refused — but this needs to be done when faced with a medically indicated situation where "the disease has won." The "naked equality of one life with another"[11] means that there is a right to equal treatment based on medical criteria without letting nonmedical criteria send us in a direction toward wrongful discrimination against those deemed too expensive or too burdensome.

Ramsey has applied his medical indications model specifically to treatment and care of imperiled newborns — and specifically in a critique of physicians letting some babies die "not only on the basis of the newborn's medical condition and prognosis, but on the basis of familial, social and economic factors as well."[12] Regardless of the economic issues at stake, Ramsey maintains that "to deliberately make medical care a function of inequalities that exist at birth is evidently to add injustice to injury and fate." To make decisions based on such social factors is "playing God," and Ramsey would at least hope that if physicians are going to do this they do so "as God plays God."[13] But as Christians, we know our God does not factor social considerations into respect for human life. Nor does our God curtail care for us based on these factors.

9. Paul Ramsey, *Ethics at the Edges of Life: Medical and Legal Intersections* (New Haven: Yale University Press, 1978), 188.

10. Ramsey, *The Patient as Person*, xvi.

11. Paul Ramsey, "The Sanctity of Life — in the First of It," *Dublin Review* 511 (Spring 1967): 10.

12. William Werpehowski and Stephen D. Crocco, eds., *The Essential Paul Ramsey* (New Haven: Yale University Press, 1994), 247.

13. Werpehowski and Crocco, *The Essential Paul Ramsey*, 248-49.

God "cares according to need, not capacity or merit." A physician's decision "to treat or not to treat should be the same for the normal and abnormal alike."[14] True humanism, Ramsey asserts, leads to an "equality of life" standard based on medical indicators and not social factors.

## Ramsey: Critique

Much of what Ramsey argues for here is correct and implied in the arguments of the preceding chapter. Surely one should never turn against the good of human life. That good is absolutely unique and inviolable and finds itself embodied. However, it does not follow from any of these considerations that it is therefore unjust to consider social factors when determining whether or not to treat an imperiled newborn. While it could be consistently argued that human dignity implies the medical indications model Ramsey offers, it could also be argued that the dignity and equality Ramsey wants to defend so strongly are more dynamic and multifaceted than his medical indications model is prepared to consider. While embodiment is central to human dignity, so is the *social situation* of that embodied person. It is precisely the *relationship* that the embodied person has with her community and her God that defines and delimits her dignity. It is certainly not "evidently" clear that, in giving lifesaving resources to one person over another, one is "turning against the good" of human life. For several hundred years the Roman Catholic moral tradition has been developing a fairly systematic way in which one can take seriously the concept of human dignity, within its total spiritual-social reality, applied to medical treatment decisions. In attempting to answer Ramsey, it is to this tradition that we turn.

## The Roman Catholic Tradition
## on Ordinary and Extraordinary Means

The distinction between a medical treatment that is ordinary and therefore morally required (in a possibly lifesaving or life-prolonging

---

14. Werpehowski and Crocco, *The Essential Paul Ramsey,* 251.

situation) and one that is extraordinary and may be refused or withdrawn, while going back at least to medieval Roman Catholic thinkers,
has been adopted (at least in some form) and invoked in the wider secular debate of these issues. However, it is important and appropriate to
get perspective on this tradition by briefly locating it in its historical
context.[15]

Many locate the beginning of this tradition's trajectory with
Thomas Aquinas's thirteenth-century attempts to balance one's abid-
ing respect for human life with some acknowledgment that the duty to
sustain such life, a temporal good, is not absolute. God has dominion
over human life, and responsible stewardship of God's gifts may mean
choosing other goods over those of human biological life. Three centuries later, moralist Francisco de Vitoria started reasoning in a way remi-
niscent of the current ordinary/extraordinary means tradition. In dealing with the question of a very sick person's refusal of food, he claimed
that if the patient is so depressed that taking food becomes "a kind of
impossibility," then the patient is not guilty of the mortal sin of suicide
— especially if there is little hope for life. Interestingly, Vitoria adds that
even if it would be more nutritious (and thus more likely to yield a
healthier state), the sick person is not required to eat the best or most
expensive food. Indeed, he broadens out this point in claiming that one
is not obliged to sacrifice one's whole means of subsistence, nor one's
general lifestyle, nor one's homeland to acquire a cure or maintain op-
timum health.

Prior to the development of modern anesthetics, surgical procedures not only involved mutilation and disfigurement of the body, but
almost always involved virtually unimaginable pain. Also in the six-
teenth century, Domingo Soto, O.P., claimed that such surgeries — and
especially amputations — were necessarily optional because of their
torturous nature. Even if medically beneficial or even lifesaving, they
could be forgone because the pain was beyond what the "common
man" could possibly be forced to bear. Though it appears that another
sixteenth-century thinker, Dominican Domingo Banez, was the first to
use the terms "ordinary" and "extraordinary" in this medical context,
Jesuit Gerald Kelly explored, summarized, and gave synthetic expres-

---

15. Most of the narrative here is owed to Richard C. Sparks, *To Treat or Not to Treat:
Bioethics and the Handicapped Newborn* (New York: Paulist, 1988), 94-100.

sion to the distinction in the mid–twentieth century. For Kelly, an ordinary treatment was obtained without very great difficulty, while an extraordinary one was obtained with excessive difficulty — with respect to pain, repugnance, cost, "and so forth." Of course, such judgments are going to depend on one's social circumstances — a particular treatment in which anesthetic is used, for instance, now could be considered ordinary whereas in the century previous it would have everywhere been considered extraordinary. Importantly, one extenuating circumstance that would make any medical means extraordinary would be if there was no reasonable hope for benefit of the patient.[16]

A few years after Kelly's work came out, Pope Pius XII delivered an address that, even though the ordinary/extraordinary distinction had appeared in the Roman Catholic moral manuals for centuries, gave it clear papal confirmation:

> Natural reason and Christian morals say that man (and whosoever is entrusted with the task of taking care of his fellowman) has the right and duty in the case of serious illness to take the necessary treatment for the preservation of life and health. . . . But normally one is held to use only ordinary means — according to circumstances of persons, places, times and culture — that is to say means that do not involve any grave burden for oneself or another. A more strict obligation would be too burdensome for most men and would render the attainment of the higher, more important good too difficult. Life, health, all temporal activities are in fact subordinated to spiritual ends. On the other hand, one is not forbidden to take more than the strictly necessary steps to preserve life and health, as long as he does not fail in some more serious duty. . . . [And] if it appears that the attempt at resuscitation constitutes in reality such a burden for the family that one cannot in all conscience impose it upon them, they can lawfully insist that the doctor should discontinue these attempts, and the doctor can lawfully comply.[17]

16. It is worth noting here that this is the "early" Kelly. Later Kelly retreats from talk about benefit to the patient. The tradition on this distinction is by no means without confusion and gray area — as we will soon see. However, this messiness does not detract from its basic premise: that human goods beyond what can be determined merely by medical indications should indeed be factored into medical treatment decisions.

17. Pius XII, "Prolongation of Life," *Pope Speaks* 4 (1958): 395-96.

To return to the first insight that called the Ramsey medical indications approach into question: "Before anything else, the doctor should consider the whole man, in the unity of his person, that is to say, not merely his physical condition but his psychological state as well as his spiritual and moral ideals and his place in society."[18]

On the basis of this history, one can come up with some general principles that characterize the ordinary/extraordinary distinction:

1. Physical life is a basic precious value that one has an obligation to protect and preserve. However, physical life is a limited value subordinated to the pursuit of spiritual ends.
2. One's moral obligation to prolong life through medical means is evaluated in light of one's overall medical condition and one's ability to pursue the spiritual ends of life.
3. One is morally obliged to prolong life with medical means when it offers a reasonable hope of benefit in helping one to pursue the spiritual ends of life without imposing an excessive burden.
4. One is not morally obliged to prolong life with medical means when death is imminent and medical treatment will only prolong the dying process; when medical treatment offers no reasonable hope of benefit in terms of helping one pursue the spiritual ends of life; or when medical treatment imposes an excessive burden on one and profoundly frustrates one's pursuit of the spiritual ends of life.[19]

---

18. Pius XII, "Cancer, a Medical and Social Problem," as quoted in Sparks, *To Treat*, 92.

19. One might wonder whether this principle still holds in light of the latest document from the Congregation for the Doctrine of the Faith, *Responses to Certain Questions of the United States Catholic Conference of Bishops on Nutrition and Hydration* (August 1, 2007). In response to the question of whether or not food and water must be provided for a patient in a persistent vegetative state (PVS) who is deemed by competent physicians to have no capacity to regain consciousness, it claims, "A patient in a 'permanent vegetative state' is a person with fundamental human dignity and must, therefore, receive ordinary and proportionate care which includes, in principle, the administration of water and food even by artificial means." Though one might ask a legitimate question about whether this answer conforms to previous church teaching, it still may be seen as consistent with principle 4. One might claim that giving a patient artificial nutrition and hydration is not medical treatment, but rather a kind of generalized "care" and therefore something that doesn't fall under the ordinary/extraordinary distinction. One

5. Benefit and burden are understood broadly in the Catholic tradition to refer not just to the physiological dimension of life, but also to the psychological, social, and spiritual dimensions.[20]

6. Cost to the individual and cost to the family are social factors that may be considered when determining whether or not a treatment imposes an excessive burden.

Much of the debate surrounding ordinary and extraordinary means has to do with complex patient-centered distinctions like those between the benefit/burden of a patient's treatment and the benefit/burden of the patient's life. While these are interesting and important issues in bioethics, the essential principle for the central issue of this chapter is #6 above. The Catholic approach here differs dramatically from the Ramsey medical indications approach in that it asks the physician to see the patient in the totality of her social reality — and in light of the spiritual and moral ideals that define and delimit her dignity and duties within that reality. These indications are far beyond *medicine's* ability to assess and imply that physicians and other health care providers need to be far more than simply highly educated technicians. If they truly have as their goal care of the person — and not just treatment of disease — then the medical indications policy falls short.

But what, specifically, does this kind of spiritual-social reasoning mean for treatment of imperiled newborns? Richard Sparks, whose thought will be examined in some detail in chapter 3, takes this question very seriously.[21] He notes that even noncompetent patients like imperiled newborns are not isolated, but rather are social creatures — members of the commonweal who are affected by the decisions of oth-

---

might also see the phrase "in principle" as an opening. For it certainly is the case that, in principle, food and water is a proportionate treatment (given the resources of most cultures) — but in some situations with less resources it might be disproportionate treatment. Also, if a PVS patient were to need other kinds of *medical* treatments (say, cardiac resuscitation), nothing in the document points to this being, in principle, ordinary treatment.

20. The preceding principles are taken from Michael R. Panicola, "Quality of Life and the Critically Ill Newborn: Life and Death Decision Making in the Neonatal Context" (Ph.D. diss., Saint Louis University, 2000), 218-19.

21. Sparks, *To Treat,* 107-13.

ers and who affect others through decisions made with reference to them.[22] As such, their proxy decision-makers may rightly factor familial and other social concerns into the ordinary/extraordinary distinction. As seen above, Pius XII included grave burden for oneself *or another* in his definition of extraordinary means. With regard to the family of the newborn, while care must be given to caution against potential greed and other selfish motives, the excessive emotional and financial strain on parents and fellow siblings is a genuine component of an infant's life situation and is certainly not inconsequential. The psychological and financial resources of a family have limits — and the strain could be enough to threaten the essential functioning of the family unit. In such cases, analogous to the case of the sick person with food or the wounded person facing amputation, treatment of the imperiled newborn might be a practical "moral impossibility" and therefore extraordinary treatment. One might think that in these situations society at large is under an obligation to provide the treatment if it is ordinary with respect to the benefit of the newborn herself. But then the next logical question — and it is a central question of this book — is, Could the (short- and) long-term costs of a handicapped infant's medical treatments and care ever be judged excessively burdensome even for society, and therefore categorically extraordinary and optional? In theory at least, the answer appears to be yes. There appears to be no theoretical reason why social factors, if they apply to treatment decisions made by the nuclear family, should not also apply to the treatment decisions of the larger family of one's society at large.[23] Just as with the nuclear family, society's resources are limited and could be strained to the point where its "essential functioning" is threatened. Though health care providers and physicians can do their best to imitate Ramsey's God, they must face the fact that we do not have the same resources.

However, to allow this kind of reasoning on such a broad scale

22. In this sense, he agrees strongly with McCormick over and against Ramsey regarding social duties of newborns.

23. This is especially true if we consider Catholic social teaching's central principle of solidarity. However, one might indeed have the practical worry about a state being motivated by expediency or corruption rather than a loving commitment to the best interest of the newborn. But this is a worry that one might have about the nuclear family as well, and is not a good reason to make a strong disjunctive move between them.

would at least allow for the possibility of far more dramatic *practical* implications than limiting it to nuclear family considerations. One could consistently argue that while certain kinds of social considerations are acceptable to consider in *theory,* in practice they could lead to such bad consequences that they should ultimately be rejected.

## Ruling Out Social Factors on a Practical Level: Richard McCormick

Foundational Roman Catholic ethicist Richard McCormick has thought quite a bit about these questions; the fact that he is sometimes difficult to follow exemplifies the wide confusion that these issues generate. On the one hand, he quite often disparages the use of the ordinary/extraordinary distinction. As far back as 1976 McCormick claimed in a *Linacre* article that he would agree that "the terms 'ordinary' and 'extraordinary' are not too helpful. They are code words for other judgments."[24] In a *Hastings Center Report* in 1978 McCormick claimed that "it must be pointed out that the terms ordinary and extraordinary are so relative that they are equally capable of abuse as quality of life language. . . . In sum, then, I would seriously question whether means language protects human life."[25] However, if one looks at his relationship with the substance of the principles of the ordinary/extraordinary distinction, it seems clear that he is largely in agreement. Consider each of the principles again and McCormick's agreement:

1. Physical life is a basic precious value that one has an obligation to protect and preserve. However, physical life is a limited value subordinated to the pursuit of spiritual ends.

"Life is indeed a basic and precious good, but a good to be preserved precisely as the condition of other values."[26]

---

24. Richard A. McCormick, "The Preservation of Life," *Linacre Quarterly* 43 (May 1976): 94.

25. Richard A. McCormick, "Quality of Life, the Sanctity of Life," *Hastings Center Report* 8 (Fall 1978): 35.

26. Richard A. McCormick, "To Save or Let Die: The Dilemma of Modern Medicine," *Journal of the American Medical Association* 229 (July 8, 1974): 174.

2. One's moral obligation to prolong life through medical means is evaluated in light of one's overall medical condition and one's ability to pursue the spiritual ends of life.

"The meaning, substance, and consummation of life is found in human *relationships*. . . . It is neither inhuman nor unchristian to say that there comes a point where an individual's [medical] condition itself represents the negation of any truly human — i.e., relational — potential."[27]

3. One is morally obliged to prolong life with medical means when it offers a reasonable hope of benefit in helping one to pursue the spiritual ends of life without imposing an excessive burden.

McCormick spends most of his time arguing about principle 4; he takes principle 3 for granted as uncontroversial. However, regarding those infants diagnosed with mental illness that still leaves room for relational potential, he says, "Life-sustaining interventions may not be omitted simply because the baby was retarded [*sic*]."[28]

4. One is not morally obliged to prolong life with medical means when death is imminent and medical treatment will only prolong the dying process; when medical treatment offers no reasonable hope of benefit in terms of helping one pursue the spiritual ends of life; or when medical treatment imposes an excessive burden on one and profoundly frustrates one's pursuit of the spiritual ends of life.

"Life sustaining intervention may be omitted when there is excessive hardship on the patient, especially when this is combined with poor prognosis."[29]

5. Benefit and burden are understood broadly in the Catholic tradition to refer not just to the physiological dimension of life, but also to the psychological, social, and spiritual dimensions.

27. McCormick, "To Save," 174 and 175.
28. Richard A. McCormick, *How Brave a New World? Dilemmas in Bioethics,* 1st ed. (Garden City, N.Y.: Doubleday, 1981), 358.
29. McCormick, *How Brave?* 358.

McCormick often builds on the personalism of Vatican Council II, which insists that human dignity be "integrally and adequately" considered.[30] This "refers to the sum of dimensions of the person that constitute human well-being: bodily health; intellectual and spiritual well-being, which includes the freedom to form one's own convictions on important moral and religious questions; and social well-being in all its forms: familial, economic, political, international and religious."[31]

Despite disparaging the use of the terms "ordinary" and "extraordinary," McCormick quite clearly supports the basic principles of the distinction looked at thus far. However, with regard to the final principle, McCormick is once again difficult to follow.

6. Cost to the individual and cost to the family are social factors that may be considered when determining whether or not a treatment imposes an excessive burden.

On the one hand, McCormick clearly supports the consideration of these social factors — at least in theory. Given his theological anthropology of the human person as "essentially social,"[32] and also what has been quoted above, it would be difficult to reject them and avoid inconsistency. Citing Catholic tradition on this question positively, he says, "if the financial cost of life-preserving care was crushing, that is, if it creates grave hardships for one or one's family, it was considered extraordinary and nonobligatory."[33] In an article he wrote for *Second Opinion*'s neonatal ethics series, he asked, "Do the sometimes staggering costs of neonatal intensive care mean that at some point the economics of care determine the meaning of best interests [of the infant]? We shy away from such considerations, and this is undoubtedly a healthy response. But how long we can sustain it I do not know."[34] He

30. Richard A. McCormick, *The Critical Calling: Reflections on Moral Dilemmas since Vatican II* (Washington, D.C.: Georgetown University Press, 1989), 156.

31. Richard A. McCormick, *Corrective Vision: Explorations in Moral Theology* (Kansas City, Mo.: Sheed and Ward, 1994), 202.

32. Again, this comes right out of Vatican Council II. See the *Pastoral Constitution on the Church in the Modern World*, nos. 12 and 32.

33. McCormick, "To Save," 174-75.

34. Richard A. McCormick, "The Best Interests of the Baby," *Second Opinion* 2 (July 1986): 21.

left the theoretical door open to consider social factors as part of the infant's good and best interest twelve years earlier in the *Journal of the American Medical Association* article,[35] but ultimately, on a practical level, McCormick refuses to walk through it. In an article he wrote with John Paris in 1983 for *America* magazine, he states rather clearly that issues surrounding life-preserving treatment of imperiled newborns "ought not be framed in terms of emotional or financial burden on the family."[36] Three years later he is just as, if not more, direct on this question: "First, lifesaving interventions ought not be omitted for institutional or managerial reasons. Included in this specification is the ability of this particular family to cope with a badly disabled baby . . . it remains an unacceptable erosion of our respect for life to make the gift of life once given depend on the personalities and emotional or financial capacities of the parents alone. No one ought to be allowed to die simply because the parents are not up to the task. At this point society has certain responsibilities."[37] More will be said later about whether or not this is an inconsistent (or, perhaps, incomplete) position based on commitments McCormick has already made. Before going there, however, we turn to John Paris, who makes a similar distinction.

## Ruling Out Social Factors on a Practical Level: John Paris

Another prominent Roman Catholic ethicist, John Paris also believes strongly in the principles espoused by the ordinary/extraordinary distinction. While he does believe that physical life is a precious value, our "ultimate goal is the restoration of the fullness of the kingdom.

---

35. "It remains then only to emphasize that these decisions must be made in terms of the child's good, this alone. But that good, as fundamentally a relational good, has many dimensions. Pius XII, in speaking of the duty to preserve life, noted that this duty, 'derives from well-ordered charity, from submission to the Creator, from social justice, as well as from devotion toward his family.' All of these considerations pertain to that 'high, more important good.' If that is the case with the duty to preserve life, then the decision not to preserve life must likewise take all of these into account in determining what is for the child's good." McCormick, "To Save," 176.

36. Richard A. McCormick and John Paris, "Saving Defective Infants: Options for Life or Death," *America*, April 23, 1983, 315.

37. Richard A. McCormick, *Health and Medicine in the Catholic Tradition: Tradition in Transition* (New York: Crossroad, 1984), 147.

Thus, it is eternal life and not life itself which is ultimate."[38] Medical indications are important, of course, but the chief end of human activity is also to be considered paramount: "simply love, the giving and receiving of love . . . a love that proves itself in the concrete world of justice, gratitude, forbearance, and charity."[39] Regarding the distinction between ordinary and extraordinary means, Paris says: "Ordinary means are those which are not disproportionately costly, burdensome or painful, and — this is the important part — they must also offer substantial hope of benefit to the patient as a person, not simply to his liver, lungs or heart. What we are to be valued for is our personhood, and if the treatment cannot offer substantial benefit to the person, not just to his or her chemistries, it is extraordinary and need not be applied."[40]

Paris has often attempted to respond to an apparent shift in Catholic teaching on artificial nutrition/hydration and ordinary/extraordinary means. Citing the New Jersey Catholic Conference of Bishops, he argues that in the limited times in which such artificial nutrition/hydration is able to be withdrawn morally, it "is designed not to hasten the death by starvation or dehydration, but to spare the patient the prolongation of life when the patient can derive no benefit from such prolongation."[41] In backing up his position he refers to the two giants in the history of the ordinary/extraordinary distinction cited above. Francisco de Vitoria argued that one was not obliged to take food if it was excessively burdensome, and if this was true in his time, "how much more so today for total parenteral nutrition, feed gastrostomies, nasogastric tubes and other artificial means of providing alimentation?"[42] He also cites Gerald Kelly, who, after a thorough survey of the prior teachings on the subject, finds that "no remedy is obligatory unless it offers a reasonable hope of checking or curing a disease."[43]

38. John J. Paris, "Terminating Treatment for Newborns: A Theological Perspective," in *Quality of Life: The New Medical Dilemma*, ed. James J. Walter and Thomas A. Shannon (New York: Paulist, 1990), 154.

39. Paris, "Terminating Treatment for Newborns," 154.

40. Paris, "Terminating Treatment for Newborns," 156.

41. John Paris and Richard McCormick, "The Catholic Tradition on the Use of Nutrition and Fluids," *America*, May 2, 1987, 358.

42. Paris and McCormick, "The Catholic Tradition," 358.

43. Paris and McCormick, "The Catholic Tradition," 359.

So Paris is largely on board with principles 1-5 detailed above — indeed, he uses them as central supports in his most important arguments. But what of principle 6, that "Cost to the individual and cost to the family are social factors that may be considered when determining whether or not a treatment imposes an excessive burden"? Like McCormick, Paris is difficult to follow on this question. It seems that he does accept these criteria on a theoretical level. We have already seen how one of his criteria for a means to be ordinary was that it is "not disproportionately costly."[44] In this same article, Paris goes on to specify the way such costs may be taken into account. After citing positively magisterial teaching that "excessive expense to the family" might make a given treatment extraordinary, he asks us to consider the case of "a 27 year old woman who fell off a horse, was decerebrate, quadriplegic, and maintained in the community hospital for some 18 years. . . . [The physicians] noted that the cost of such care would be astronomical, almost beyond belief. Well, if one calculates at a very low rate of $300 a day, and builds in an inflation factor of 12 percent, 18 years of such care comes to $6,104,590. The Vatican reaffirms the duty of physicians to take such factors into account."[45] This is a remarkable point for at least two reasons. First, considering that the article was written over twenty-five years ago, the number — already astounding — would be that much more dramatic given today's costs. Second, Paris speaks affirmatively of a *duty* to take such broad social factors into consideration. This becomes all the more remarkable when one considers other things he has written on this subject.

Paris wrote the article with McCormick that claimed that treatment of imperiled newborns "ought not be framed in terms of the emotional or financial burden on the family."[46] In the *Quality of Life* volume, Paris, when considering whether or not the financial or emotional burdens could truncate an infant's right to life, answers with "an emphatic 'no.'"[47] He claims that "although parents may continue to be involved in decision making for their children, they do not have the sole right to demand or refuse medical interventions for the infant. It is the child's best interest, not the parent's wishes, that is to govern treatment deci-

---

44. Paris, "Terminating Treatment for Newborns," 156.
45. Paris, "Terminating Treatment for Newborns," 158.
46. McCormick and Paris, "Saving Defective Infants," 315.
47. Paris, "Terminating Treatment for Newborns," 152.

sions."[48] He makes the same point even more strongly in a letter to the editors of *Law, Medicine and Healthcare:* "I wish to join those who raise their voice against the theory that children are to be accepted or rejected — to live or be killed — because of their burden on others. . . . It is the interest of the patient, and the harm to the patient, which have been and ought to be the primary focus of medical ethics. To deviate from that norm is to distort if not destroy medicine's role in society."[49]

## Ruling Out Social Factors on a Practical Level: Magisterial Teaching

The reasoning of some members of the magisterium — and especially that of the United States bishops — mirrors that of McCormick and Paris. The Congregation for the Doctrine of the Faith's *Declaration on Euthanasia,* for instance, claims that refusal of treatment out of "a desire not to impose excessive expense on the family or the community" is "considered as an acceptance of the human condition."[50] However, while the United States Catholic Conference of Bishops (USCCB) claims that "in principle cost can be a valid factor in decisions about life support" (for example, money spent on expensive treatment for one family member may be otherwise needed for food, housing, and other necessities),[51] they also claim that, while the problem "requires further study and discussion," what "is best for the individual child should take precedence over any conflicted interests of parents or society" — and the solution to this problem is "increased local, state and federal assistance" to families that find themselves in this situation.[52] The Pennsylvania Catholic Bishops add that, given the society in which we live, the argument that social factors should be considered (at least

48. John Paris, "Parental Discretion in Refusal of Treatment for Newborns," *Clinics in Perinatology* 23 (September 1996): 575.

49. John Paris, "Letter to the Editors: Handicapped Infants and Their Families," *Law, Medicine and Healthcare* 11 (October 1983): 231.

50. Congregatio pro Doctrina Fidei, *Declaration on Euthanasia* (Washington, D.C.: Publications Office, United States Catholic Conference, 1980), 12.

51. United States Catholic Conference of Bishops (USCCB), "Nutrition and Hydration: Moral and Pastoral Reflections," *Origins Online* 21, no. 44 (1992).

52. National Conference of Catholic Bishops: Committee for Pro-Life Activities and American Jewish Congress, "Treatment of Handicapped Newborns" (July 26, 1985).

with regard to the family) is "not convincing" because "resources are available from other sources and these can often be tapped before a family reaches dire financial straits. Such assistance has been and continues to be available."[53]

## McCormick, Paris, and Magisterial Teaching: Critical Evaluation

A quick read of McCormick, Paris, and the American bishops[54] on these issues can be difficult to reconcile — and some might even be tempted to call their views self-contradictory. On the one hand, they seem to accept, and accept rather strongly, the principles behind Catholic teaching on ordinary and extraordinary means — including those regarding the application of social issues in making the distinction. On the other hand, each makes very clear that social factors should not determine treatment decisions regarding life-prolonging therapies for imperiled newborns. What is going on here? Richard Sparks attempts to shed some light on this issue by arguing that while in *theory* "McCormick, Paris, et al. are willing to consider familial and social 'costs' in determining the burden component related to prolonging life, ultimately their fears of potential abuse lead to non-inclusion or at least a tendency toward exclusion of such social burden factors."[55] This seems especially true for McCormick — who seems to fear abuse on two levels. "First he fears that a broad interpretation of social factors can easily lead to the slippery slope of social utilitarianism. This, he understands, can lead to infanticide. Second, McCormick is well aware of the finite and sinful nature of humanity. How does one determine if a family is taking the never-competent patient's perspective or their own self-interested perspective?"[56] In addi-

---

53. Pennsylvania Catholic Bishops, *Nutrition and Hydration: Moral Considerations* (1999).

54. It should be noted that the teaching under critical evaluation is that of the United States bishops — but not the Roman Congregation for the Doctrine of the Faith. The latter does not make the theory/practice distinction in the documents cited.

55. Sparks, *To Treat*, 179.

56. Peter A. Clark, *To Treat or Not to Treat: The Ethical Methodology of Richard A. McCormick, S.J., as Applied to Treatment Decisions for Handicapped Newborns* (Omaha: Creighton University Press, 2003), 216.

tion, Sparks wonders if McCormick and Paris don't take social factors into consideration more than one might think at first glance. He says, "it is not clear whether McCormick and Paris absolutely exclude all social burden factors."[57] For, in their joint paper in *America,* they point to the fact that the family shouldn't be allowed to discontinue *because society can absorb the cost* — but then they neglect to speculate on whether the cost of an imperiled newborn's treatment ever exceeds a society's duty to treat her.[58]

Though Sparks and Clark are helpful here, this doesn't get these views off the hook with regard to the charge of inconsistency. Let us take the theory/practice distinction and the worry about potential abuse. First, it is not clear that incorporating social factors, especially when disciplined by the Catholic moral tradition's principles beyond the ordinary/extraordinary distinction,[59] will indeed lead down a slippery slope toward bad things like social utilitarianism. Indeed, one could certainly approach social factor inclusion from the *patient's* perspective rather than society's interests. Also, Catholic social teaching demands that we approach social factor inclusion with *distributive justice* in mind — not social utility. Second, it is not clear, even if something like a social calculus were used, that infanticide would be (or even would likely be) the result. We currently use a (often poorly conceived) social calculus in determining how community monies are spent in public health programs like Medicare and Medicaid — this kind of reasoning has not led us closer to things like infanticide.[60] Indeed, whatever arguments lead to the conclusion that infanticide would be the likely result of social quality of life reasoning also lead to the conclusion that infanticide would be the likely result of more traditional quality of life reasoning. For, even when working with a strict "best interest"[61] quality of life model —

57. Sparks, *To Treat,* 199.

58. Sparks, *To Treat,* 200.

59. The classic distinction between acting directly against the good of human life and letting die as a foreseen and unintended consequence, for instance. Also see Clark on the many other safeguards that exist in this tradition, including McCormick's relational quality-of-life criterion itself. Clark, *To Treat,* 216.

60. Though this goes well beyond the scope of this book, it is worth noting here that social calculus might specifically *preclude* systematic active euthanasia of imperiled newborns due to the callousness and disrespect for life that would result.

61. Later in the chapter, a possible distinction between a "strict" model of best in-

through which it was determined that the burdens of a particular life-prolonging treatment outweighed the benefits — one could certainly have the worry that infanticide, being more direct, cost-effective, timely, and (arguably) less painful than withdrawal or refusal of treatment, would be the result of slippery-slope reasoning. If a view accepts the social quality of life model "in theory but not practice" because it might lead to infanticide, it should reason the same way about the strict "patient best interest" quality of life model as well — one which all three above accept.

But what about Sparks's suggestion that perhaps McCormick and Paris's model is not that strict after all? Perhaps they offer an opening to consider social factors by claiming that families should not be allowed to discontinue treatment because, in part, society can pick up the tab. Might the *way* society picks up the tab be subject to the considerations of the social quality of life model? The central argument of this book is "surely yes," but that conclusion is difficult to come to given the direct commitment of McCormick to not consider "institutional and managerial" reasons for discontinuing treatment of an imperiled newborn and Paris's scolding those who support factoring in the interests of others as contributing to the "destruction of the role of medicine in society." The USCCB explicitly rejects this move by claiming that "decisions about life-extending care should not be determined by macro-economic concerns such as national budget priorities and the high cost of healthcare. These social problems are serious, but it is by no means established that they require depriving chronically ill and helpless patients of effective and easily tolerated measures that they need to survive."[62] This might be the way to go as an argument independent of McCormick, Paris, and the American bishops — but as a matter of internal consistency they appear to be forced to reject it.

In continuing a critique of these positions, it is helpful to consider the theological and moral anthropology in play. Each of the three to a certain extent, but McCormick perhaps most dramatically, holds a strong *relational anthropology*. He thinks the social nature of human be-

---

terests (one that would include only the isolated, individual interests of the person) and a "broad" model (one that would include the interests of a patient specifically situated in the patient's social context) will be explored.

62. USCCB, "Nutrition and Hydration."

ings is present even in nonvolitional newborns. Paris locates the essential value identity of human life in loving relationships. And Catholic social teaching's theological anthropology starts with the human person as she exists "in social relationship." It is difficult to see, then, how each can hold such an anthropology that is so dramatically connected to a social context — and yet rule out social considerations on a practical level when deciding how best to respect the dignity of human life in imperiled newborns. As Sparks articulately notes: "McCormick's absolute declaration that decisions 'must be made in terms of the child's good, this alone' does not itself forestall incorporating some social factors as they relate to the infant's holistic well-being. For that matter, his advocacy of relational potential as the measure of the infant's minimal interest in life-saving treatment is a family-oriented, socially-conscious criterion, at least as viewed from the patient's perspective."[63] And:

> In their admirable effort to avoid a socially-weighed bias against a patient's own experience of burden vis-a-vis benefit, I believe the more restrictive quality of life proponents have construed the determination of excessive burden too narrowly. The ultimate decision as to whether treatment is in a given patient's total best interest ought to incorporate not only medical or individualistic (i.e., experimental) burden factors, but also broader social factors, viewed from the patient's existentially-contexted vantage point. On this level, the broader interpreters of the quality of the patient's life echo the best of the ordinary/extraordinary tradition in their insistence that the cost, psychic strain, and degree of inconvenience borne by others, a non-competent's social network, ought rightly to be factored in as part of the patient's burden, holistically considered.[64]

A final argument for rejecting the theory/practice distinction involves the *absolutely overwhelming* injustice and need when it comes to medical resources. Health care is the single most expensive component of our nation's budget (and, especially in light of health care reform, the arrow continues to point up). Such monies are allocated not primarily on the basis of need or justice, but in large part according to a market profitability scheme and political considerations. The profit-

63. Sparks, *To Treat,* 180.
64. Sparks, *To Treat,* 198.

ability of treating NICU patients dramatically and unjustly skews how community money is spent on the nation's poor. That such radical and far-reaching injustice exists is a strong reason to reconsider legitimate worries about a slippery slope — especially in light of previous concerns.

Despite what appears to be the U.S. bishops arguing the contrary, the resources to meet every medical need of our families, under our current (or any) health care system, simply do not exist — at least if we want to justly allocate resources as a culture. If we truly take Ramsey seriously that medicine is about the "good of human beings," then we must take these numbers seriously and practically — not just theoretically. Paris himself seems to be arguing this very point when he calculates the cost of a patient's treatment at a very low rate of $300 a day, with an inflation factor of 12 percent, and finds that eighteen years of such care comes to $6,104,590. "The Vatican reaffirms the duty of physicians to take such factors into account."[65] How can Paris argue what appears to be a self-contradictory position here — namely, that taking into account the cost to others is to distort if not destroy medicine's role in society and that physicians have a duty to take cost into account?

Panicola suggests one route in his treatment of Paris's position. He says that from reading him "one might get the impression" that "Paris fits better into the narrow social quality of life camp." This, he claims, "is the wrong impression" because Paris is claiming that social factors may be considered for patients only when the "life-sustaining treatment provides no benefit to *them*, and it is a careless use of resources to sustain their lives when they receive no meaningful benefit."[66]

Does this work for the case in which Paris explicitly argues for taking social considerations into practical account? Well, he does claim that the patient is "decerebrate" — which, depending on whether this refers to a neurological state or a bodily posture, could be the kind of human being that Panicola insists that Paris is talking about. At the very least, Paris does not justify his consideration of social factors by arguing that the patient could not have benefited from the treatment anyway. But let us say for the sake of argument that Panicola is correct. Does this still keep Paris out of the social quality of life camp?

65. Paris, "Terminating Treatment for Newborns," 158.
66. Panicola, "Quality of Life," 157.

In answering this question one should consider seriously the arguments of Joseph Boyle in his article "A Case for Sometimes Tube-Feeding Patients in Persistent Vegetative State."[67] Boyle argues that the claim that treatment of PVS (and like) patients is of no benefit needs to be called into serious question. He admits that "by any estimate, the benefits of keeping a person alive who has no prospect of recovering from . . . radically impaired consciousness . . . are small." However, such patients "can be harmed by being killed, by being treated as spectacles or sex objects, by being used improperly for experimental purposes and so on." And, if such indignities are harms, "then actions taken precisely to prevent or remove these indignities must be benefits to them."[68] But what about the burdens of treatment? "The pain, suffering and interference with the pursuit of valued activities which often provide reasons for discontinuing treatment are not possible for [a] patient in PVS,"[69] and many of these kinds of burdens are also not possible for others with similarly impaired consciousnesses. Therefore, Boyle argues, most of the time the burdens involved in the treatment of such patients "must be those imposed on others."[70] In the case that Paris presents to us, the burdens imposed on others are astronomical — and would, given Boyle's argument, probably be enough to tip the balance in favor of nontreatment. However, the reason behind it would not be the one Panicola suggests — it is not that treatment of the patient provides no benefit to *her,* but rather that treatment's burden to others is so large that it overrides what little benefit it does give the patient with radically impaired consciousness. But this is precisely the argument of the social quality of life model. Now, in fairness to Panicola, Paris may believe that such treatment does not benefit the patient and thus remain consistent. However, if Boyle is correct, the set of those with radically impaired consciousnesses — such that they cannot benefit from treatment — is very small indeed.

67. Joseph Boyle, "A Case for Sometimes Tube-Feeding Patients in Persistent Vegetative State," in *Euthanasia Examined: Ethical, Clinical, and Legal Perspectives,* ed. John Keown (Cambridge: Cambridge University Press, 1995), 189-99.

68. Boyle, "A Case," 192-93.

69. Boyle, "A Case," 194.

70. Boyle, "A Case," 195.

## Wrongful Discrimination?

Arguments against the social quality of life model might take a different track from the ones considered so far. One might claim, for instance, that taking into account social factors when deciding whether or not to treat imperiled newborns is de facto wrongful discrimination. Someone who has made this argument quite forcefully is John Arras. In his article "Toward an Ethic of Ambiguity,"[71] he freely admits that some "nonmedical" problems may seem attractive, at first glance, for consideration when making treatment decisions about newborns. For instance, parents may "face the dilemma of keeping their child at home, where the demands of caring for her disabilities are likely to drain their economic and emotional resources, or handing her over to an institution that is likely to be underfinanced and understaffed." Even though "socially induced burdens can join forces with strictly physical disabilities," Arras claims that nevertheless "we must base our treatment decisions solely on the extent of medical disabilities. To take social factors into account is to act unjustly toward the child." He puts the point more bluntly: "To say that the wealthy child should live (because her anomalies are not so severe as to make life too burdensome) but that the poor child with similar prognosis should die (because of further burdens imposed by her poverty) is to indulge in the rankest kind of discrimination."[72] Indeed, we should avoid "morally dubious justifications based on the well-being of other interested parties, such as parents, siblings, or even of society at large."[73]

J. H. M. Dorscheidt, a Dutch legal scholar, wrote a book in which he explored the connection between the Dutch policy of deliberate termination of the lives of certain imperiled newborns and international law prohibiting discrimination against the disabled — specifically, against children with regard to medical care.[74] Dorscheidt argues that the Dutch policy violates both explicit and implicit international law — citing documents like the UN Children's Rights Convention and

71. John D. Arras, "Toward an Ethic of Ambiguity," *Hastings Center Report* 14 (April 1984): 25-33.

72. Arras, "Toward an Ethic," 27-28.

73. Arras, "Toward an Ethic," 26.

74. J. H. M. Dorscheidt, *Levensbeeindiging Bij Gehandicapte Pasgeborenen: Strijdig Met Het Non-Discriminatiebeginsel?* (The Hague: SDU, 2006).

the UN Convention to Promote and Protect the Rights and Dignity of Persons with Disabilities. The UN Convention on the Rights of Persons with Disabilities[75] claims, "'Discrimination on the basis of Disability' means any distinction, exclusion or restriction on the basis of disability which has the purpose or effect of impairing or nullifying the recognition, enjoyment or exercise, on an equal basis with others, of all human rights and fundamental freedoms in the political, economic, social, cultural, civil or any other field" (article 2). Later, when speaking specifically of "children with disabilities, the best interests of the child shall be a primary consideration" (article 8, section 1). With regard to health, the convention claims that "persons with disabilities have the right to the enjoyment of the highest attainable standard of health without discrimination on the basis of disability," and that persons with disabilities should have "the same range, quality and standard of free or affordable health care and programmes as provided to other persons" (article 25, section a). The UN Children's Rights Convention[76] also weighs in on this issue, claiming that "a mentally or physically disabled child should enjoy a full and decent life, in conditions which ensure dignity, promote self-reliance and facilitate the child's active participation in the community," and that nation-states "shall encourage and ensure the extension, subject to available resources, to the eligible child and those responsible for his or her care, of assistance for which application is made as which is appropriate to the child's condition and to the circumstances of the parents or others caring for the child" (article 23, sections 1 and 2). However, if one wishes to convincingly argue that "taking into account social factors when deciding whether or not to treat an imperiled newborn" is wrongful discrimination against the disabled, further clarification is demanded; specifically, two concepts need to be better defined: disability and discrimination.

What does "disability" mean in this context? A disability is any medical or psychological malady that *substantially limits one or more of the*

75. United Nations General Assembly, "Convention of the Rights of Persons with Disabilities" (December 6, 2006); http://www.un.org/esa/socdev/enable/rights/convtexte .htm (accessed September 15, 2007).

76. Theresia Degener and Yolan Koster-Dreese, *Human Rights and Disabled Persons: Essays and Relevant Human Rights Instruments,* vol. 40 (Dordrecht and Boston: M. Nijhoff, 1995), 198-225.

*major life activities of an individual.*[77] Does a supporter of the social quality of life model necessarily discriminate on the basis of disability so defined? The answer appears to be no. The model is not concerned with disability in this sense, but rather with how social factors — like financial (and other) costs to the family and broader community — should be considered in determining whether a treatment is burdensome or beneficial. It might often happen that someone with a disability has the costs and burdens factored in such that social factors will be strong considerations. Indeed, the subjects of each of our four case studies from chapter 1 certainly would appear to fall into this category. However, one could certainly think of a case in which the social quality of life model would take social factors into consideration in which the patient was *not* disabled in the narrow sense. Consider someone with significant heart disease such that if he does not have bypass surgery and take expensive medicines he will likely have a massive heart attack and die. However, until that time his life will be basically normal and he will be able to engage in all the life activities that he wishes. One could certainly argue, using the social quality of life model, that the social factors surrounding the burden to his family and community should be considered in determining whether or not he should get this treatment — without wrongfully discriminating against a disabled person. If this sense of disability is correct, then the claim that invocation of social factors is "the rankest kind of discrimination" against the disabled is simply false.[78] Indeed, this is why the subject of this book is "imperiled" newborns rather than "disabled" newborns. It is a meaningful and important distinction to make.

But let us suppose that a more broad sense of disability is the correct one. Though it certainly strains common sense to think of disabil-

---

77. This is the definition of the U.S. Equal Employment Opportunity Commission. United States Equal Employment Opportunity Commission, "Section 902: Definition of the Term Disability"; http://www.eeoc.gov/policy/docs/902cm.html (accessed September 15, 2007). Perhaps one could define disability more broadly as "any medical or psychological malady" at all. But this would seem to violate the commonsense meaning of the term, which is generally connected to a malady that impairs one or more life activities of an individual.

78. One still might consider the prospect that it wrongfully discriminates on the basis of access to resources. This is something that will be taken up in some detail in the book's final chapter.

ity as a physical or mental malady that does not affect a life activity,[79] let us suppose for the sake of argument that all who are subjects of nontreatment under the social quality of life model are in fact disabled. Does it follow that the social quality of life model is *wrongfully discriminating* against the disabled? Though this move would put Arras, Dorscheidt, and company on stronger ground, the answer is still no. The key here is to define precisely what one means by "discrimination." In a later article,[80] Arras is quite concerned with defining this idea and suggests that rising from the ashes of the political fight over Baby Doe[81] were three possible definitions of "discrimination" in this context:

1. Discrimination is failure to provide customary care, or the appropriate "standard of care," for newborn infants.
2. Discrimination is failure to provide care to a disabled child that would have been provided to an otherwise normal child.
3. Discrimination is denying medical benefits to a disabled child solely on the basis of the infant's present or anticipated disability.

The first definition cannot be the correct one because the reason this topic is controversial is that no "customary" care or "standard of care" exists with regard to the controversial cases in question. Or, perhaps better, simply invoking "standard of care" with regard to controversial cases in the gray area has the practical effect of begging the question. If there was agreement about the standard in these cases, we would not be debating this issue at all.[82]

The second definition is more convincing — and would seem to work in many cases. It certainly works for the case of Baby Doe, in which she

79. Or perhaps one need not think of present disability as the only relevant kind. Perhaps someone who is facing a future death from a heart attack is "disabled" in the sense that he may be dead before he is able to engage in the kinds of activities he wants to: witnessing his children's weddings, grandchildren's baptisms, etc.

80. John Arras and Nancy Rhoden, "Withholding Treatment from Baby Doe: From Discrimination to Child Abuse," *Milbank Memorial Fund Quarterly* 63 (Winter 1985): 18-51.

81. Arras is primarily concerned in this section of the article in critiquing the senses in which the U.S. Department of Health and Human Services defined "disability" in order to respond to the Baby Doe case and make sure disabled infants would not get "discriminatory" medical treatment or nontreatment.

82. Arras and Rhoden, "Withholding Treatment," 24.

was diagnosed with a problem with her esophagus, but also with Down syndrome — and lifesaving treatment was rejected, but only because of the genetic disability. Everyone seems to see this as wrongful discrimination on the basis of disability. However, the disability and the medical problem requiring treatment (blockage of the esophagus) are separable in a way that makes this judgment work. It is not always the case. Consider an infant born with a meningomyelocele (failure of the neural tube to develop during fetal life, causing part of the spine to be exposed) accompanied by hydrocephalus (an abnormal buildup of cerebral spinal fluid that, in this case, will likely cause mental retardation). Arras argues that it is meaningless to ask the question, "Apart from the child's hydrocephalus and possible retardation, would we seal up the spinal column of an 'otherwise normal' baby?" He claims that while we may certainly wish to close the spine, we cannot exclude the accompanying difficulties from our consideration. If we choose to operate, we choose to do so based on the best interests of the child — and not because we would perform the operation on an "otherwise normal" child.[83]

Arras argues that the third definition, "rather than any well-thought-out moral theory of discrimination," is rather a "philosophical rejection of quality of life reasoning" — and this is evidence that the trappings of nondiscrimination and of civil rights law appear merely to have served as convenient vehicles for advancing a narrow "sanctity of life" agenda.[84]

But if none of these work, what *is* discrimination in our context? In a general sense, as Arras notes, discrimination is not immoral: it is simply to make distinctions between two or more things or persons. Wrongful discrimination is not merely making distinctions that result in unequal treatment. For, when "a distinction is based on a relevant trait, there is no discrimination; but when people are treated differently solely on the basis of irrelevant criteria, then we have genuine discrimination."[85] What kind of discrimination, then, is the social quality of life model using? It seems clear that, even if we assume the dubious broad definition of disability, the basis on which the model discriminates has nothing *directly* to do with disability at all. Rather, the model

83. Arras and Rhoden, "Withholding Treatment," 25.
84. Arras and Rhoden, "Withholding Treatment," 26-27.
85. Arras and Rhoden, "Withholding Treatment," 27.

discriminates on the basis of social cost to the family and community. Such a model is noncommittal about whether or not one could ever discriminate on the basis of disability: its discrimination takes place with regard to the treatment cost to a patient's family and community, not whether or not a patient is disabled or whether her individual quality of life makes it "worth living." The social quality of life model bypasses these questions altogether and does not discriminate on the basis of disability.[86] It does, of course, discriminate on the basis of a treatment's cost to a family or society — and it seems clear that Arras would consider this to be an "irrelevant" basis for discrimination. However, he does not give an argument for this point of view, and might do well to heed the clause inserted into the point made by the UN Children's Rights Convention that subjects our duties to treat disabled children "to the availability of resources."

The social quality of life model does not discriminate wrongfully against the disabled. All persons (disabled or not) have a right to a proportionate amount of the community's resources — and a duty to refrain from using a disproportionate amount.

## The Social Quality of Life Model and "The Moral Foundations of Medicine"

Michael Panicola fires another volley at the social quality of life model by, again, calling it out for basing treatment decisions on familial and social factors rather than patient-centered factors. He argues that one should not rely on predictions about the cost of treatment to a family or on the burdens imposed on society — rather, the main concern should be the newborn's good, and this alone. This means that external factors should be left out of the decision-making process.[87] If they

---

86. Even if the social quality of life model is not discrimination against the disabled in the sense that disability is not the basis by which it discriminates, one might still argue that it is de facto discrimination against the disabled because a majority of babies not treated have disabilities. This move gets into complex questions about wrongful discrimination's relationship to an act's intention versus its consequences — but suffice to say here that difficult decisions must be made in a situation where needs dramatically outstrip resources. More on this in the final chapter.

87. Panicola, "Quality of Life," 162.

enter explicitly into life-sustaining treatment decisions for imperiled newborns, he argues (much like Paris) that this "poses a serious threat to the moral foundations of medicine." Panicola explains:

> Traditionally, the patient-practitioner relationship has focused on the individual patient in need with a tendency toward excluding external factors. While a fair amount of latitude has been given to patients in assessing the burdens imposed on others within this relationship, the main emphasis of the practitioner has always been on the patient's best interests. The social quality of life approach would have practitioners refocus their sights to include the interests of affected others. This would certainly undermine the sacred trust upon which the patient-practitioner is founded. Consequently, patients and proxy decision-makers would be left wondering whose good or interests the practitioner is promoting.[88]

We can say at least two things about this argument. First, someone could certainly support the social quality of life model such that social factors were explicitly considered in treatment decisions of imperiled newborns on the level of *managed* care within a particular health care financer — like Medicaid or a private insurance company. This is happening already — and it does not necessarily involve the explicit decision of a practitioner in a specific clinical setting. Rather, social factors are considered at a prior level and take the form of rules and regulations over which the practitioner has little or no control. Thus, the physician would be able to make treatment decisions with the best interests of the patient in mind — but within a set of rules and regulations that are sensitive to social factors with which the physician has nothing to do. Second, we need to return to moral anthropology here. If one accepts that a human person is essentially social, then distinguishing between a physician having "her" good or the good of "affected others" in mind is a questionable move. If one takes the broader Catholic understanding of relational anthropology seriously, there is no such thing as good "for her" in the individual abstract — without reference to the good of affected others. Indeed, for a physician to pretend otherwise is to engage in anthropological self-deception. One's good is always connected to the good of affected others — at least if one

---

88. Panicola, "Quality of Life," 110.

is living in a community. And a physician is bound to accept this regardless of what the history of medicine has been. A physician should indeed focus on the "best interests" of the individual patient in need — but those interests go far beyond medical indications of an individual person's biological body. They include that person holistically considered — her spiritual and social realities are to be considered primary indicators when it comes to treatment decisions.

But Edmund Pellegrino builds on Panicola's argument — in ways that challenge my response.[89] He claims that the modern age has brought with it tremendous confusion about the role and identity of medicine. "Is the physician still a helper, healer and caregiver? Or are physicians something else — gatekeepers, guardians of society's resources and employees, 'managed' by gag rules and restrictive clauses, or entrepreneurs and co-investors in commerce of healthcare?"[90] Pellegrino suggests that there is something internal to medicine itself, something inherent in its nature as a particular human activity, which does not allow it to be set upon externally by some form of social construction — relative to the values of a culture. On the one hand we have the "essential" *ends* of medicine — that which gives it an essential character. They grow out of the phenomenology of medicine: "the universal experience of illness." This experience transcends time, place, history, and culture — and identifies objective ends that are to be contrasted with socially constructed *goals* that "open medicine to possible subversion by economics, politics, social ideology or government."[91] Whenever "medicine is used for any purpose or goal — however defined — that distorts, frustrates, or impairs its capacity to achieve its proper ends, it loses its integrity as a craft and its moral status as a human activity. . . . We have socially crucial reasons for maintaining the internally defined ends of medicine. Without ends, there is no source of criticism, no counter to the most malevolent uses of power of medical knowledge and skill by individuals, societies or governments."[92]

---

89. Edmund D. Pellegrino, "The Goals and Ends of Medicine: How Are They to Be Defined?" in *The Goals of Medicine: The Forgotten Issue in Health Care Reform*, ed. Mark J. Hanson and Daniel Callahan (Washington, D.C.: Georgetown University Press, 1999), 55-68.

90. Pellegrino, "Goals and Ends," 55.

91. Pellegrino, "Goals and Ends," 60.

92. Pellegrino, "Goals and Ends," 64.

But how do these considerations relate to an evaluation of the social quality of life model? Pellegrino admits that "physicians are members of the moral community" and as such have obligations "to advocate just distribution of physicians, healthcare resources, and facilities. A role of advocacy in distributive justice is a collective moral obligation of physicians."[93] But these fall under the category of societal goals — and, as such, must be "second" to the internal ends of medicine. When a physician is

> serving the end of medicine as medicine, the physician's focus must be his covenant with his patient. The physician is then bound by a covenant of trust which must not be compromised by other roles of, for example, the physician as gatekeeper, entrepreneur, guardian of social resources, or by the economic pressures to undertreat. . . . The welfare of the patient, jointly determined between physician and patient or patient's morally valid surrogate must continue to be the end of medicine in the clinical encounter and first in the order of priorities for the physician's role.[94]

Though Pellegrino's argument is intuitively convincing, there are several questions to ask. The first is about internal consistency. Pellegrino is at pains to show that the internal ends of medicine cannot be trumped by the mere goals of society. But why? There are "socially crucial" reasons for keeping medicine's internal ends unassailable — this permits us to critique those who would use the power of medicine for "malevolent" purposes. But how is one supposed to determine what a "malevolent" purpose is without appealing to the kinds of social "goals" that Pellegrino says are never more basic than the ends of medicine? Sure, the ends of medicine may speak of the covenant between the patient and the physician — but this, by itself, is not enough to condemn the Nazi-like practices he invokes. For these the central issue is the moral status of certain human beings and whether or not they count as patients in such a covenant. To condemn such medical practices, one is going to have to appeal to — at least as Pellegrino defines it — mere societal goals like, say, respecting the moral status of all human beings. But this is precisely what cannot be

93. Pellegrino, "Goals and Ends," 66.
94. Pellegrino, "Goals and Ends," 65.

the case if Pellegrino is correct. Supposedly contingent societal goals cannot be the reason for keeping medicine's ends unassailable, for, if they were, then as these goals shift and change, so would the status of medicine's ends.

Second, we pose a counterexample to the assertion that the internal ends of medicine are wrongfully distorted when a physician violates the supposed covenant between her and a patient by allowing economic considerations or distributive justice to be considered. What should one think of the triage or battlefield medic? Clearly, her role is to distribute her resources (in this case, the time she has to treat wounded soldiers) in a just way — and this sometimes means meeting, often face-to-face, with patients and then sometimes passing them by, realizing that even though they could be saved by spending significant resources, she could save more lives by moving on to someone else. Here is a clear example of, according to Pellegrino, a supposedly mere societal goal (distributive justice) trumping what is supposedly an internal end of medicine (the patient/physician covenant). Pellegrino would seem to have to reject this — but it is unclear where his complaint would be lodged. The medic has done nothing wrong and, to the contrary, would be *unjust* if she spent undue time on the first patient she met — based on a supposed physician/patient covenant — with the result that several others died who could have otherwise been saved. One can pose the battlefield medic as a counterexample without arguing that any current clinical situation is analogous to that of a battlefield. Though chapter 3 will argue that such an analogy is convincing in some important situations, all one needs here for a counterexample is *any* situation in which a physician acts correctly in factoring distributive justice concerns ahead of a supposed physician/patient covenant. Surely the battlefield medic counts as just such a physician — and a heroic one at that.

A third question surrounds Pellegrino's consideration of matters of economic concern and distributive justice to be mere "goals" of society (changeable and malleable) rather than just as fundamental to, and a legitimate end of, medicine as treatment and care of patients. This builds on the original response given to both Ramsey and Panicola: that of relational anthropology. One's social relations — and duty to exist in just relationship — are intrinsic aspects of the patient. Indeed, if there is a patient/physician covenant, then it is to the patient *holisti-*

*cally considered* that a physician has a duty. The ends of medicine surely do include, at a primary level, treatment and care of patients — but built essentially into these ends must be the restriction that treatment and care is just to others that are affected by it; this cannot be meaningfully considered without taking social factors into consideration.

## Can Imperiled Newborns Have Duties?

The last paragraph spoke of a "duty to exist in just relationship" being an essential part of what it means to be a human being. But how can this be said of the imperiled newborn? It certainly appears that such nonvolitional human beings have no moral duties at all — and thus perhaps duties connected to social relationships should not be considered when it comes to treatment of imperiled newborns. Such is the argument of Paul Ramsey in his article "Enforcement of Morals: Nontherapeutic Research on Children."[95] Though the article is about proxy consent for experimentation on children, the piece's key issue is the issue at hand: moral duties of nonvolitional children. Ramsey notes that to impute consent (and, by extension, moral duties) to a child "is to treat a child as not a child. . . . It is to treat him as if he were an adult person." With regard to the social quality of life model, Ramsey would say that it is immoral to assume children have any social duties with regard to distributive justice because they "cannot themselves consent" to such duties and "ought not be presumed to consent."[96] The good of living in just relationship may be intrinsic to a volitional adult, but it is not a good for the imperiled newborn. As yet, the imperiled newborn "is not a moral agent, not a bearer of moral obligations, even presumptive ones."[97]

Richard McCormick responds to Ramsey in his "Experimentation in Children: Sharing in Sociality." McCormick asks us to recall the reason why any consent from parents for medical treatment for their infant is valid: "precisely insofar as it is a reasonable presumption of the

95. Paul Ramsey, "Enforcement of Morals: Nontherapeutic Research on Children," *Hastings Center Report* 6 (August 1976): 21-29.
96. Ramsey, "Enforcement of Morals," 21.
97. Ramsey, "Enforcement of Morals," 25.

child's wishes." He then argues that behind the finding that the child "would wish" something is the conviction that the child *ought* to wish it. There are "things that the child *ought*, simply as a human being, to choose." He grants Ramsey's point that infants have no actual moral obligations, "but the language of *ought* need not imply actual obligations."

> If we can say of adults (who can and do have obligations) that it is reasonable to expect that they will want certain goods for others and contribute to these goods if there is discernible risk, discomfort, or inconvenience, it is not precisely because they are adults that we conclude this, but *because they are social human beings*. Being adults we assume that they will understand, acknowledge, and respond to the claims rooted in their sociality, their social nature. And we call the *experience* of such claims an *ought*. But the claims themselves are rooted in the sociality of our being. They are not primarily rooted in the adult's capacity or willingness to respond to them as an adult . . . but in the social nature of human beings. Now this sociality is shared quite as much by infants as by adults. *Ought* language is but an attempt to highlight this. That is, in using such language the focus is sociality, not age. The good of infants is inseparably interlocked and interrelated to the good of others; for they are human beings. Clearly, they cannot experience this or respond to its implications as claims. But we may for them — to the extent that it is reasonable to do so, a reasonableness founded on their common share in our human nature.[98]

McCormick suggests that the root of their disagreement may come from (once again) their differences over theological anthropology — and claims that Ramsey has a "narrowly individualistic notion of human nature." Certain kinds of moral duties are not predicated on individualistic ideas about volitionality or consent. Rather, they are predicated on the nature of human beings as intrinsically social and are binding regardless of whether consent is offered or not — or capable of being offered or not. Indeed, as Pope Benedict XVI reminds us in his latest encyclical, *Caritas in Veritate*, "rights presuppose duties" and "individual rights, when detached from a framework of duties which

98. McCormick, "Experimentation in Children," 42.

grants them full meaning, can run wild."[99] Many persons, including newborn infants, have rights that, because they are incapable of consent, must be defended by proxy. They therefore have presupposed duties that must also be acted on through some kind of proxy agent as well.

Ramsey responds to McCormick[100] somewhat begrudgingly — and with some amazement that McCormick offers the argument he does: "The charge is that I 'hold a narrowly individualistic notion of human nature' and believe an incompetent patient to be 'an unrelated reality.' 'Isolationism' is the verdict. If an 'individualist' is one who believes a child is not *born* with sociality in exercise, then I am one."[101] But this misses the point. Sociality is not something that is necessarily "exercised" — rather, it is an essential part of the nature of all human beings.[102] We are participating in it regardless of whether or not we are aware of it or choosing it, or capable of being aware of it or choosing it. It is a strange thing for Ramsey to argue against, because at times he appears to be making exactly this kind of argument. In his extended thinking about "covenant" between God and humanity — and between human beings — he claims that human beings exist in covenant from the beginning: "A man is never without his fellow man in any such fashion, nor does he reach his neighbor only by choice or contract from which he can as easily withdraw. Instead, because his creatureliness is from the beginning in the form of fellow humanity and because the creation in him is in order to covenant, and because this means he has real being only by *with* and *for* fellow man, we have to reckon with this in everything that is said about justice and about the rights of man."[103] It appears that he and McCormick are not that far apart after all.

99. Benedict XVI, *Caritas in Veritate* (2009), 43; http://www.vatican.va/holy_father/benedict_xvi/encyclicals/documents/hf_ben-xvi_enc_20090629_caritas-in-veritate_en.html (accessed August 10, 2009).

100. Paul Ramsey, "Children as Research Subjects: A Reply," *Hastings Center Report* 7 (April 1977): 40-42.

101. Ramsey, "Children as Research Subjects," 40.

102. One might wonder how this is possible if we are to take seriously the idea that human infants are persons simply because they are human organisms. But recall the argument from the first chapter: it is not simply being a human organism that carries the moral weight; rather, it is the natural potential of that organism for certain morally relevant capacities — like relationality.

103. Werpehowski and Crocco, *The Essential Paul Ramsey,* 115.

Like the "medical indications" discussion that began this chapter, the key point here is one of theological and moral anthropology. If one is convinced of the intrinsically relational anthropology, and therefore the intrinsically social nature of human beings, then the arguments like this against the social quality of life model fall flat.[104]

## A Postscript on Relational Anthropology: A Necessary Ingredient in the Social Quality of Life Model?

Much of this chapter has attempted to show how important a relational anthropology is for responding to the charge that medicine needs to always be in the best interest of the individual patient. It is worth very briefly noting that though many beyond the Catholic Church have a relational anthropology, one need not accept it to accept the social quality of life model. A relational anthropology becomes important in the context of avoiding the charges of undermining individual human dignity or the covenant between physician and patient. If one wants to keep the sole focus of the physician and health care system on the individual and still accept the social quality of life model, then relational anthropology becomes indispensable. But one could certainly persuasively argue, as James McCartney does, that not all limitations and restrictions of care must be based in the infant's "questionable ability to benefit [broadly conceived] from this treatment, but on the sheer fact that it may cost too much, may involve personnel who are needed elsewhere, [and] may utilize resources that could more readily save many more lives. . . . While I agree that we ought to do all we can to mitigate these factors, when they are irrevocably present I hold that they would provide adequate justification for the foregoing or discontinuance of treatment."[105]

104. This chapter makes no argument about how, precisely, social factors are to be taken into consideration either theoretically (as primary or secondary factors) or practically. These questions are answered in chapters 3 and 4.

105. James McCartney, "Issues in Death and Dying," in *Moral Theology: Challenges for the Future* (Mahwah, N.J.: Paulist, 2003), 279.

# CHAPTER 3

# The "Weak" Social Quality of Life Model

*The ordinary/extraordinary means tradition ushered in the possibility of expanding the notion of the patient-person and of his/her best interests to include such social components as cost and burden to affected others, but always as subsidiary elements of the patient's interests.*

Richard Sparks[1]

To this point we have looked at two kinds of approaches to the social quality of life model. The first approach accepted the model in its "strong" version — which claims that social factors should have a primary, rather than secondary, importance when making treatment decisions regarding imperiled newborns. That approach was shown to have been founded on a faulty moral anthropology. Because even the most imperiled newborn is a person, and because this approach relied on the premise that such newborns are not persons, it was found to be unconvincing. The second approach attempted to show that, because even the most imperiled newborn is a person, the social quality of life model — in whatever form — violates human dignity in a theoretically and/or practically unacceptable way. However, this approach is also founded on a faulty moral anthropology. Because the concept of human dignity does not and cannot exist apart from social relationship, and therefore

1. Richard C. Sparks, *To Treat or Not to Treat: Bioethics and the Handicapped Newborn* (New York: Paulist, 1988), 273.

social duty, social factors must play some kind of role in deciding whether or not to treat an imperiled newborn. What we have not explored is just *how much weight* should be given to social factors and *on whom* the social factors should focus. This chapter explores a "weak" version of the social quality of life model — an approach that, while accepting the necessary place social factors play in treatment decisions, sees them as secondary rather than primary considerations and factors that apply only to the narrowly considered best interests of the newborn and not to the broader ground of the interests of affected others. Arguments to this effect from Raymond Duff and A. G. M. Campbell, Paul Johnson, Anthony Shaw, and Richard Sparks will be considered.

In response to this approach, the central argument of the book will be brought to bear — critiquing the "weak" version of the social quality of life model in light of Catholic social teaching. A central flaw will again be found in the moral anthropology of the approach in that it underestimates just *how* connected human dignity is to social considerations — something that cannot be argued for more strongly in the Catholic social tradition. They are not essential but merely secondary considerations, but rather essential and *primary* considerations. In addition, the approach underestimates just how overwhelming the social factors at stake actually are — not just for NICU care, but for follow-up care and education as well. This affects not only the families directly involved, but also the resources available for other departments in clinics and hospitals, those under Medicaid and private insurance, and, to a significant extent, our national health care system. The argument that this is analogous to a "triage" situation — which, by definition, includes social factors with regard to distribution of resources (time, money, etc.) as primary considerations — will be evaluated with particular reference to Medicaid. Though the chapter's last section will examine several good reasons to be skeptical of the triage analogy, it will conclude that, with so much at stake, the idea that social factors are only of secondary importance is untenable.

## Raymond Duff and A. G. M. Campbell

Duff and Campbell have written several articles (both jointly and individually) from the "weak" social quality of life perspective. They claim that when making treatment decisions with regard to an imperiled newborn's best interests, the relevant facts and circumstances that one should consider are the infant's "future health, development, and well-being, and the human costs that are likely to accrue with survival."[2] The concept of "human costs" is, however, rather vague and requires further definition. Duff and Campbell claim that the "rights of patients to live or die and the rights of family members and others in the present and future generations must be considered."[3] A choice for treatment might be "bad" if "the parents have little or no capacity to care for their child, where the family does not want to be forced to do what they believe should not be done and where resources to help the child or the family are limited or absent."[4] Though they are very open about the explicit and direct role that social factors should play, it is clear they intend to argue that they should be taken into consideration only when it serves the child's narrowly conceived interests.

> Since one cannot prudently ignore the family's limitations and interests even if considering only the child's interests, responsible decision makers cannot avoid the "tragic choices," that is, at times knowingly sacrificing, perhaps unfairly, one person's good or life in order to protect another's. With a sense of balance, irony, and tragedy it is understandable, right, and common that the family's interests are sacrificed to the benefit of the child. With a similar sense, the converse may be true particularly when the child may benefit little even though the family sacrifices much.[5]

Though social factors are to be considered, the individualistically narrow interests of the infant are still to take precedence — for it is really only when a child cannot directly benefit "much" from a treatment that social factors can trump. Indeed, the only time parents' decisions for or against treatment can be overridden is when they "select a

2. A. G. M. Campbell, "Quality of Life as a Decision-Making Criterion I," in *Ethics in Perinatology,* ed. Amnon Goldworth et al. (New York: Oxford University Press, 1995), 83.

3. John Ladd, *Ethical Issues Relating to Life and Death* (Oxford: Oxford University Press, 1979), 201.

4. A. G. M. Campbell and R. S. Duff, "Authors' Response to Richard Sherlock's Commentary," *Journal of Medical Ethics: The Journal of the Institute of Medical Ethics* 5 (Spring 1979): 141.

5. Raymond Duff, "Counseling Families and Deciding Care of Severely Defective Children: A Way of Coping with 'Medical Vietnam,'" *Pediatrics* 67 (March 1981): 316.

course which goes too far toward sacrificing their child's interests and seeking their own."[6]

## Anthony Shaw

Physician Anthony Shaw's "weak" version of the model comes directly out of his experience as a physician working with imperiled newborns. He says that for years he simply accepted that treatment decisions should be focused on the newborn's "mental and physical capacity," but eventually came to the conclusion that if more factors are not considered then something important has been neglected. Indeed, one must consider "aptitudes, motivation, skills and pleasure, physical and intellectual, which the individual acquires as a result of efforts made on his behalf by his *family* and by *society*.."[7] Shaw gives a simple mathematical formula to illustrate how this might be done.

QL = quality of life
NE = infant's natural endowment (physical and mental)
H   = support from the infant's home/family
S   = support from society

He says his old view — and the view (like Ramsey's medical indications model) of those who reject even the weak version of the social quality of life model — is:

$$QL = NE$$

However, the formula *should* look like this:

$$QL = NE(H+S)$$

Considering only the objective natural endowment of the infant misses the fact that such a natural endowment exists not in a theoretical vacuum, but in a social situation that directly affects quality of life. Even if

6. Duff, "Counseling Families," 28.
7. Anthony Shaw, "Defining the Quality of Life," *Hastings Center Report* 7, no. 5 (October 1977): 11. All quotations and citations from Shaw in the next few paragraphs are from page 11 of this article.

the natural endowment is well above zero, the quality of life depends, in large measure, on what social resources are available to support an imperiled newborn — enhanced in certain situations where the family or society provides support, and diminished if they do not. Notice that where there is zero social support the objective natural endowment is meaningless and therefore QL = 0. If this formula is correct, it is a good indicator that the concept of QL in any nonsocial sense is a misguided one.

Shaw, like Campbell and Duff, makes it clear that what is at stake when considering social factors are the individualistically narrow interests of the newborn — which should be separated from consideration of the newborn's impact on the family and society. When applying his formula to a newborn with Down syndrome, he is at pains to show that the social factors he considers (including the extent to which the parents have the emotional and financial resources to give all the care that is necessary) "all influence the quality of life *of the baby*." Indeed, he makes it clear again and again that proper application of the formula "excludes potential contributions to or detractions from society and family when considering any individual's potential quality of life."

## Paul Johnson

Paul Johnson is largely in support of the formula offered by Shaw — and builds directly upon it. He says we are dealing with a medical culture with a bias toward preserving life. And Christians, particularly those convinced by the tradition of the ordinary/extraordinary distinction, should be careful about such bias — especially "given the lack of accessibility to sufficient assistance to all families and given the competition for scarce monetary and manpower resources in society."[8] A bias like this is not necessarily bad, but "such a commitment to life logically should entail commitment to provision of means to support and enhance life."[9] It is not fair to choose life for a newborn "and not choose to allocate the resources

---

8. Paul R. Johnson, "Selective Nontreatment of Defective Newborns: An Ethical Analysis," in *On Moral Medicine: Theological Perspectives in Medical Ethics,* ed. Stephen E. Lammers and Allen Verhey, 1st ed. (Grand Rapids: Eerdmans, 1987), 497.

9. Johnson, "Selective Nontreatment of Defective Newborns," 496.

to make that life livable."[10] Families who care for these children need the assistance of special education, physical therapies, and family counseling. Financial relief and respite care may be necessary. Institutions for raising such children need to be fully funded and staffed so as to be genuinely compassionate rather than simply give custodial care. Given the enormous costs associated with such a commitment, "Severe strain and dislocation can be brought on families. And minimal provision of resources may not be sufficient to assure extensive and adequate care."[11] While Johnson admits that ethical and medical decisions ought not to simply reflect often unjust social structures, "neither ought they be made without any reference to them. Recognizing that financial and personnel resources are not inexhaustible, allocation decisions will have to be made and consequences faced honestly."[12]

Johnson offers us the same warning as the authors cited above. When considering social factors, "The further one proceeds from the immediate burden placed on the infant . . . the more caution is called for."[13] If one starts with the personhood of the infant (as all authors outside of chapter 1 do), then "Respect for the person should lead to criteria established with the best interest of the infant, not society, in mind."[14] Rather than doing a utilitarian calculus, we must give "specific concern primarily to the best interests of the infant."[15] Johnson acknowledges that "costs have traditionally played some role in the determination of some means of life preservation as extraordinary and therefore elective," while also arguing that "societal and parental resources are important to the degree that lack thereof affect the future well-being of the infant."[16] Without this individualistically narrow focus on social factors as they impact the best interests of the infant, he maintains, we are left "open to great abuse" and also "might override the newborn's right to life."[17] Interestingly, because of "even currently

10. Johnson, "Selective Nontreatment of Defective Newborns," 499.

11. Johnson, "Selective Nontreatment of Defective Newborns," 497.

12. Johnson, "Selective Nontreatment of Defective Newborns," 499.

13. Johnson, "Selective Nontreatment of Defective Newborns," 497.

14. Paul Johnson, "Selective Nontreatment and Spina Bifida: A Case Study in Ethical Theory and Application," *Bioethics Quarterly* 3 (Summer 1981): 99.

15. Johnson, "Selective Nontreatment and Spina Bifida," 103.

16. Johnson, "Selective Nontreatment and Spina Bifida," 98.

17. Johnson, "Selective Nontreatment and Spina Bifida," 97, 103.

available societal and family support resources," Johnson believes that "quality of life consideration in ordinary-extraordinary analysis is to be more restrictive than permissive of nontreatment."[18]

We can formulate at least three principles common to all the thinkers considered so far:

1. Human beings are indeed intrinsically social creatures.
2. Intrinsic sociality means that one cannot consider the best interests or quality of life of the newborn without considering social factors that impact on her best interests and dignity.
3. However, social factors can only impact treatment decisions based on *how those factors impact the newborn's best interests,* considered from an individualistically narrow point of view.

This is certainly a logically consistent way of interpreting both the intrinsic sociality of the human person and the essential place social factors have in considering whether or not a treatment is ordinary or extraordinary — both essential characteristics of the social quality of life model. However, though the mistake of the above thinkers is not as fundamental as that of the thinkers considered in chapter 2, it is cut out of the same cloth. It is also a mistake of moral anthropology. We have discussed Richard McCormick's specific argument for the fundamental sociality of the human person in the context of arguing for the social duties of newborns, but have only hinted at how this teaching is argued for and developed within Catholic social teaching.

## Catholic Social Teaching on the Fundamental Sociality of the Human Person

Sadly, Catholic social teaching (CST) has a reputation in some circles as being the church's "best kept secret." And to the extent that this is true (I do think CST needs a much wider audience),[19] many readers

18. Johnson, "Selective Nontreatment and Spina Bifida," 107.

19. It has been my experience that CST has an influence and plausibility that transcend political, ecclesial, and even theistic boundaries. It has the possibility of uniting liberals and conservatives, Christians and non-Christians, and theists and nontheists in very important ways.

might not be familiar with it. What is Catholic social teaching? In many ways, CST has quite ancient roots. Its central principles, like the duty to have a particular focus on the poor, certainly go back to Jesus himself — and many go back to the even more ancient Jewish traditions that also focus on the poor. But the specifically social aspects of the teaching reached another level of importance in the fourth century and beyond when Christianity became formally interconnected with the state and had responsibility for forming social policy. But in most cases, and generally in the context of this chapter, Catholic social teaching "refers to a limited body of literature written in the modern era that is a response of papal and episcopal teachers to the various political, economic and social issues of our time."[20] Though the beginning of the formal tradition seems to be a new move to emphasize "the social questions" starting with Pope Leo XIII's *Rerum Novarum* in 1891, there is no official list of documents that "count" as CST. Kenneth Himes points out: "Clearly, the expression CST is elastic, sometimes designating an expansive body of material and at other times used in a more constricted sense. . . . Perhaps we can understand the term *Catholic Social Teaching* as an effort by the pastoral teachers of the church to articulate what the broader social tradition means in the era of modern economics, politics and culture."[21]

The church's positions on abortion and euthanasia are far more commonly referenced (by Catholics and non-Catholics alike) than its social teachings, but CST should not be thought to have any less normative weight in Roman Catholic moral theology. Indeed, the last two popes explicitly referred to it as Catholic social *doctrine.*[22] Finally, though many aspects of church teaching are directed at an audience wider than explicit Catholics, the later documents of CST (starting with Pope John XXIII in the 1960s) are explicitly directed at an audience consisting of "all those of good will."

Catholic social teaching's starting point is nicely summarized thusly:

20. Kenneth R. Himes and Lisa Cahill, *Modern Catholic Social Teaching: Commentaries and Interpretations* (Washington, D.C.: Georgetown University Press, 2005), 5.

21. Kenneth R. Himes, *101 Questions on Catholic Social Teaching* (Mahwah, N.J.: Paulist, 2001), 5.

22. Pontificium Consilium de Iustitia et Pace, *Compendium of the Social Doctrine of the Church* (Dublin: Veritas, 2005), 172; hereafter Pontifical Council, *Compendium.*

The right to the common use of goods is "the first principle of the whole ethical and social order" and "the characteristic principle of Christian social doctrine" . . . it is innate in individual persons, in every person, and has *priority* with regard to any human intervention concerning good, to any legal system concerning the same, to any economic or social system or method: "All other rights, whatever they are, including property rights and the right of free trade must be subordinated to this norm [the universal destination of goods]; they must not hinder it, but rather expedite its application."[23]

Todd Whitmore has spent considerable time studying the social encyclicals of the popes who have contributed to the church's social doctrine. In writing on them,[24] Whitmore has argued on multiple occasions that one should start with the common good in Catholic social teaching because "of the repeated claim that human beings are fundamentally social."[25] The claim that human beings are somehow individually autonomous is a fiction — for "a supportive set of interrelationships is a precondition for human life and concomitant with it."[26] This is what Pope Leo XIII meant when he said man "cannot, if dwelling apart, provide himself with the necessary requirements of life, nor procure the means of developing mental and moral faculties. Hence it is divinely ordained that he should live his life — be it family, or civil — with his fellow man."[27] Two generations later, Pope Pius XI confirmed both the claim and its theological underpinning. Human persons are "endowed with a social nature." Indeed, "God has destined" them for civil society.[28] This was true from the first groups of human persons onward, but it has per-

23. Pontifical Council, *Compendium*, 82.

24. His chapter "Catholic Social Teaching: Starting with the Common Good" appears in Kathleen Maas Weigert and Alexia K. Kelley, *Living the Catholic Social Tradition: Cases and Commentary* (Lanham, Md.: Rowman and Littlefield, 2005) and makes many of the following arguments, but I will be using the following unpublished paper, which makes the arguments in more detail: Todd David Whitmore, "Catholic Social Teaching: A Synthesis" (January 14, 2004).

25. Whitmore, "Catholic Social Teaching," 5.

26. Whitmore, "Catholic Social Teaching," 6.

27. Leo XIII, *Immortale Dei* (New York: Paulist, 1941), 3.

28. Pius XI, *Quadragesimo Anno, Encyclical Letter on Reconstructing the Social Order* (Washington, D.C.: National Catholic Welfare Conference, 1942), 118, and Pope Pius XI, *Divini Redemptoris* (New York: Paulist, 1930), 29.

haps never been more dramatically true than in the modern globalized world. For "the interdependence of national economies has grown deeper, one becoming progressively more related to the other so that they become, as it were, integral parts of one world economy."[29] This was one of Vatican II's main themes — one of the "signs of the times" being that "a man's ties with his fellows are constantly being multiplied."[30] Pope John Paul II would later claim that "the church's social doctrine focuses especially on man as he is involved in a complex network of social relationships within modern societies."[31] Most recently, Pope Benedict has taken special care to recognize "that the human race is a single family working together in true communion" and that "a new trajectory of thinking is needed in order to arrive at a better understanding of the implications of being one family."[32]

In addition to being empirically true, the above claims have a theological underpinning that has been developed far beyond a simplistic claim that "God has made it this way." Human dignity, even when mistakenly considered in an autonomous fashion, is often tied to the theological claim that human persons are made "in the image of God." However, "the social documents stress that the *imago Dei* ('image of God') doctrine is precisely about image of the *triune* — that is, interrelational, God."[33] Relationality is an essential aspect of the divine nature — and, insofar as human persons share in this nature, an essential aspect of our nature as well. John Paul II says persons in society are in "the *living image* of God the Father, redeemed by the blood of Jesus Christ and placed under permanent action of the Holy Spirit. . . . This supreme *model of unity,* which is a reflection of the intimate life of God, one God in three Persons, is what Christians mean by the word *communion*."[34] Whitmore notes that Vatican II reminded us that Jesus prayed to the Father "that all may be one . . . as we are one" (John 17:21), and

29. Whitmore, "Catholic Social Teaching," 7.

30. Vatican Council II, *Gaudium et Spes* (Washington, D.C.: National Catholic Welfare Conference, 1976), 6.

31. John Paul II, *Centesimus Annus* (Washington, D.C.: Office for Publishing and Promotion Services, United States Catholic Conference, 1991), 54.

32. Benedict XVI, *Caritas in Veritate* (2009), 53.

33. Whitmore, "Catholic Social Teaching," 7.

34. John Paul II, *Sollicitudo Rei Socialis* (Washington, D.C.: Office of Publishing and Promotion Services, United States Catholic Conference, 1988), 40.

this implies a certain similarity between the union of the divine persons and the union of human persons. It reveals that man cannot fully find himself except through a sincere gift of himself.[35] It means that, as Whitmore puts it, "there is no human dignity apart from the dignity we all have in relation to each other."[36]

Whitmore goes on to argue that this concept of what one might call the "social dignity of the human person" implies a moral and sometimes legal obligation of mutual assistance. As John Paul II reminds us, our fundamental sociality means a duty to the common good, which in turn means that *"all* really are responsible for *all."*[37] Though Catholic social teaching defines the common good variously, one particularly good definition was offered at Vatican II: "the sum of those conditions of social life which allows social groups and their individual members relatively thorough and ready access to their own fulfillment."[38] One primary way that Catholic social teaching, especially when offered by John Paul II, attempts to articulate just how human persons are to live in accord with the common good is by invoking "solidarity." John Paul II says that solidarity

> is above all a question of interdependence, sensed as a system determining relationships in the contemporary world, in its economic, cultural, political, and religious elements, and accepted as a moral category. When interdependence becomes recognized in this way, the correlative response as a moral and social attitude, as a "virtue," is solidarity. This then is not a feeling of vague compassion or shallow distress at the misfortunes of so many peoples, both near and far. On the contrary, it is a firm and persevering determination to commit oneself to the common good.[39]

Solidarity can surely benefit members of the community of human persons, but it also "imposes a duty"[40] on human persons. This duty needs to be particularly aware of a "vast and unfair distinction in the

---

35. Vatican Council II, *Gaudium et Spes,* 24.
36. Whitmore, "Catholic Social Teaching," 8.
37. John Paul II, *Sollicitudo Rei Socialis,* 38.
38. Vatican Council II, *Gaudium et Spes,* 25.
39. John Paul II, *Sollicitudo Rei Socialis,* 38.
40. Paul VI, *Populorum Progressio* (1967), 17.

distribution of goods" that cannot be "in harmony with the designs of an all-wise creator."[41] Distributive injustice is also a major concern for the social teaching of Paul VI and John XXIII, who warn us respectively that "imbalance is on the increase" and that when "the wealth and conspicuous consumption of a few stand out" human rights are ineffective and "the fulfillment of duties is compromised."[42] This kind of inequality denies persons the ability to participate fully, and sometimes at all, in the institutions that constitute the communities of human persons.

In response to this inequality, one's duty is not simply to treat everyone "equally." Especially in light of Pope Benedict's reminder that "One of the deepest forms of poverty a person can experience is isolation,"[43] we must acknowledge that "equality is not an end in itself, but has value only insofar as it enables groups and persons to participate in the life of the community."[44] Paul VI says that rather than aim at noncontextualized equality, "the more fortunate should renounce some of their rights so as to place their goods more generously at the service of others."[45] A duty to what Whitmore calls "solidarity-informed egalitarianism"[46] means that there exists a "serious obligation which binds each and every one to lend mutual assistance to others" in their efforts to participate in society.[47]

In fulfilling such a duty, "it is not enough to draw on the surplus goods"[48] when lending assistance to others. Indeed, Catholic social teaching claims that one's ownership of private property, while certainly a right, might need to be given up in light of the "universal destination of goods" — the idea that all property is to be used ultimately in service of the common good of all. Indeed, one's private property is "under 'social mortgage,' which means that it has an intrinsically social function, based upon and justified precisely by the principle of the universal destination of goods."[49] Whitmore nicely summarizes still more examples:

41. Pius XI, *Quadragesimo Anno,* 64-65.
42. Paul VI, *Populorum Progressio,* 8, and John XXIII, *Mater et Magistra* (1961), 69.
43. Benedict XVI, *Caritas in Veritate,* 53.
44. Whitmore, "Catholic Social Teaching," 32.
45. Paul VI, *Octogesima Adveniens* (1971), 23.
46. Whitmore, "Catholic Social Teaching," 33.
47. John XXIII, *Pacem in Terris,* 87.
48. John Paul II, *Centesimus Annus,* 35.
49. John Paul II, *Sollicitudo Rei Socialis,* 42.

Leo states, "Man should not consider his outward possessions his own, but as common to all," and goes on to insist that "it is one thing to have a right to a possession of money, and another to have a right to use money as one pleases." Pius XI continues this line of thinking, and the Second Vatican Council cites Thomas Aquinas to take it even further. If the "universal destination of created goods" means that material goods at the level of basic need are indeed rights, then what appears to be theft from the rich by the destitute is actually legitimate. "If a person is in extreme necessity, he has the right to take from the riches of others what he himself needs." Paul VI clarifies this point by quoting the early church father, Ambrose, who insists that such actions are not theft because the goods were properly the poor person's in the first place. Therefore, when the well-off give to the poor, Paul VI tells the former, "You are not making a gift of your possessions to the poor person. You are handing over to him what is his. For what has been given in common for the use of all, you have arrogated to yourself." Put another way, "you" are the thief.[50]

Whitmore concludes that there are limits on how much of one's income and wealth one uses for one's own living — the rest belongs to the common good. If one has earned wealth one has done so partly by one's own initiative and work, but also a globalized society has created the conditions for the possibility of such work and has needs that rightly generate strict duties for us to fulfill. Indeed, one has a right to one's wealth insofar as one has needs that are part of the common good — but one does not have a right to use one's wealth in a way that violates, *or is disproportionate with,* the common good. One has a duty to use resources proportionately.

But what is the relative status of this duty? Perhaps, though real, it is a secondary duty or something that could be easily trumped by other, more primary duties. Hardly. Pius XI speaks of this duty as a "grave precept" that goes back to the Church Fathers.[51] The World Synod of Bishops declared this duty to be one of "absolute justice."[52]

50. Whitmore, "Catholic Social Teaching," 45, citing Leo XIII, *Rerum Novarum,* 19; Pius XI, *Quadragesimo Anno,* 45-49 and 56; Second Vatican Council, *Gaudium et Spes,* 69; and Paul VI, *Populorum Progressio,* 23.

51. Pius XI, *Quadragesimo Anno,* 50.

52. Synodus Episcoporum, *The Synodal Document on the Justice in the World* (Boston: St. Paul Editions, 1971), 70.

One of the most striking examples of the gravity of this duty comes from Vatican II's positive citation of the Church Father Gratian, who says, about an instance of neglect of this duty, "Feed the man dying of hunger, because if you do not feed him you have *killed* him."[53] Though Catholic moral theology is sometimes known for making a strong distinction between the gravity of active and passive actions that result in death, this does not appear to be the case where one's social duty is concerned. Indeed, to call the neglect of it "killing" means it is about as serious as a duty gets.

Recall, then, the third principle of authors espousing a "weak" social quality of life model:

> However, social factors can only impact treatment decisions based on *how those factors impact the newborn's best interests,* considered from an individualistically narrow point of view.

Can this point of view be sustained in light of what has just been presented? It seems not; for it is not only an empirical fact that human persons are *fundamentally and intrinsically* social, but this is backed up theologically by the triune, relational image of God that exists in each person. This sociality is so fundamental that one cannot speak of the "dignity" or "best interests" or "quality of life" of a human person except with reference to some kinds of social considerations.[54] But these considerations must not ultimately be forced back to an individualistically narrow moral anthropology — as the authors above try to do. The fundamental sociality of human persons "imposes a social duty" on us as well — a duty to the common good with particular reference to the "vast and unfair distinction in the distribution of goods." Such a duty requires us to limit the use of our financial and other resources such that it is proportionate with the

53. Vatican Council II, *Gaudium et Spes,* 69, emphasis added.

54. Catholic social teaching seems more comfortable using "human flourishing" or "human goods" in this context. But more often than not the book will use human *interests* instead. As mentioned previously, what is in a person's interest (especially if we take into account the moral anthropology of CST) is going to be something much broader than what one merely *prefers* — and thus this concept gets at the thick account of flourishing/goods that CST is after. It also has the added advantage of being the term used by several of the proposed interlocutors of this book and thus contributes to the possibility of conversation with them.

common good. Failure in such a duty is of the utmost seriousness — on a par with taking human life.

## Problems with Prioritizing the Common Good and the Universal Destination of Goods

One may certainly have legitimate worries about this starting point and emphasis. Indeed, if we start with the common good and universal destination of goods, don't we run the probable risk of subsuming the inherent and irreducible dignity of the human person into a social calculus of what is best for the greatest number — say, what will cause the most human flourishing? Although most ethical systems will have questions to answer on where they fall on this scale and why, Catholic social teaching's emphasis on the common good is always disciplined by other moral principles — including that certain acts cannot be ordered to God or the common good because they directly act against an intrinsic good. One cannot for any reason intend to kill an innocent person, for instance, because that acts directly against the intrinsic good of an individual human life. This is different, of course, from justly allocating resources in such a way where one will foresee, but not intend, that human lives will be lost. In the former case, the church teaches, the object of one's act is directed against human life, but in the latter case the object of one's act is just distribution of resources.

Another worry might involve the relationship between the private and public spheres in Catholic social teaching — especially for safeguarding the realm of freedom with regard to one's private property and one's social duties. The church teaches that "Private property and other forms of private ownership of goods 'assure a person a highly necessary sphere for the exercise of his personal and family autonomy and ought to be considered as an extension of human freedom.'"[55] Indeed, "Private property is an *essential* element of an authentically social and democratic economic policy, and it is the guarantee of a correct social order."[56] If this level of personal freedom with how an individual and family decide to use their resources is "highly necessary" and even

55. Pontifical Council, *Compendium*, 84.
56. Pontifical Council, *Compendium*, 84.

"essential," then can Whitmore and this book make the strong claims about the duties present in starting with the common good and the universal destination of goods? The answer is yes:

> Christian tradition has never recognized the right to private property as absolute and untouchable. "On the contrary, it has always understood this right within the broader context of the right common to all to use the goods of the whole of creation: the right to private property is subordinated to the right to common use, to the fact that goods are meant for everyone." . . . *Private Property, in fact, regardless of the concrete form of the regulations and juridical norms relative to it, is in its essence only an instrument for respecting the principle of the universal destination of goods; in the final analysis, therefore, it is not an end but a means.*[57]

Though there is an important right to freedom with regard to one's private resources, it is only an instrumental right for a more fundamental right: proportionate access to resources available for, and belonging to, the common good.

## Richard Sparks: A Rejoinder

Sparks has written an entire book explicitly dealing with the above issues: both in a survey of the literature and in forming his own argument.[58] Because his argument is the most developed of the authors considered in the first part of this chapter, and also because his is the closest to the central argument of this book, significantly more space will be given to its explication.

Sparks shares much with Catholic social teaching's understanding of the human person. At several points in his book he advocates a "holistic concept" of the human infant patient and of her best interests. He criticizes those who describe the infant's best interests "too narrowly to the physical reality of a pumping, living human organism" (269). Those who operate under a social quality of life model must widen the scope

57. Pontifical Council, *Compendium*, 84.
58. Richard C. Sparks, *To Treat or Not to Treat: Bioethics and the Handicapped Newborn* (New York: Paulist, 1988), 337. In-text page references in this section are to this work.

of a patient's best interest to include psychological, spiritual, and social factors. Indeed, to "isolate a newborn patient as if s/he is a monad wholly unrelated to family, society, and their incarnate limitations is to create an ahistorical, unreal setting for decision making" (269).

Such a conclusion leads Sparks to be in sympathy with the central argument of this book — at least on one level. He says, "Macro-allocation questions concerning budgetary priorities in light of the limits of global resources lead to valid ethical questions concerning whether any patient, generically-speaking, has a right to soak up an inordinate and unjust share of healthcare dollars, talent and energy" (269). This question, though "largely unexplored," is one that Sparks supports asking. However, it "prescinds from and prefaces actual medical practice." He claims a subtle but important distinction between socially weighting the benefit/ burden analysis (which, he admits, Roman Catholic teaching on ordinary/extraordinary means supports) on the macro-allocation level of public policy and suggesting the same method for "bedside/cribside decision making." The former is perfectly legitimate and "may well be the best moral course" (271-72) for attempting to incorporate distributive justice into health care resource-allocation decisions. However, once we enter the "intrasystem" arena of actual medical practice, this kind of socially weighted benefit/burden calculus "becomes a dangerous threat to the integrity, personhood, and rightful place that has always been reserved for the individual sick or handicapped patient in need" (273). Sparks points out that the Hippocratic oath mentions that a physician comes to a house "for the benefit of the sick" — no mention is made of the conflicting interests of the patient's family. He also mentions that the ordinary/extraordinary distinction has "ushered in the possibility of expanding the notion of the patient-person and of his/her best interests to include such social components as cost and burden to affected others, but always as *subsidiary elements* of the patient's interests, holistically considered, never as distinctive counter-claims" (273). He is simply adamant that "the EXCLUSIVE focus in actual medical practice and related decision making has heretofore always been on the best interest(s) [of the individual patient], however broadly defined. To shift that focus toward a socially-weighted calculus in which the patient's rightful interests are merely one component among a series of presumably equal counter-claims is to undervalue the primacy of the patient and to potentially discriminate against his/her rights and best interests" (273).

Like the previous authors in support of a "weak" version of the social quality of life model, Sparks legitimizes attempts to incorporate social factors like familial stress and financial limits "from the patient's perspective." Anything else opens the door to denigration of neonatal patients in the name of "pure social utility" — particularly because these patients are not competent to defend their own interests. If it were so, then the slippery slope will have been greased "toward bias against and abuse of those patients least able to assert their rights and needs in the decision making debate." In addition, he asserts that those who are all too quick to do a socially weighted calculus for newborns "tend to shun" the same reasoning for competent patients (274-75). Because of this double standard, changing the centuries-old tradition of medicine away from patient cure and care, and the denigration of the inherent personhood and inalienable rights of the disabled and noncompetent patients, "one should reject" a socially weighted calculus model "on the treatment/nontreatment decision-making level" (276).

Sparks does develop a positive argument about how to proceed at this decision-making level. Provided that one takes respectful caution against too facile a reason, he says that "it seems fair to incorporate financial and emotional costs associated with one's treatment, at least *as a correlative factor* in computing net burden related to the patient's own well-being" (298-99, emphasis added). This, of course, is with the proviso that social factors are seen as they impact on the patient's own objective and experiential best interests, not as factors stacked over and against the patient. The idea that in burdening one's own family one could also be a burden to oneself might "tip the scales" in favor of nontreatment.

How would this work in a practical situation? Sparks asks us to consider a severely handicapped nondying infant with almost no conscious relational potential. If the treatment of such a neonate would totally bankrupt one's family or contribute to a parent's probable mental breakdown or deprive a number of needy patients with far better prognoses of lifesaving medical resources, "it is possible that the patient's *total* best interests — including psychological, social and spiritual well-being — might be better served by non-treatment." Such a high cost to one's caretakers, or fellow NICU residents, may constitute too much burden for too little medical and experiential benefit. Sparks is clear that he is not advocating a socially weighted calculus "in which the interests of a newborn *with a reasonably good prognosis* can be over-ridden by social factors, but rather a patient-centered calculus, in which social factors may compound against an already negative prognosis" (301, emphasis added).

Sparks, then, gives us two methodological principles to use when attempting to incorporate social factors into the treatment of imperiled newborns. First, we can openly adopt a socially weighted, common-good-oriented calculus on the level of public policy. On the basis of studied and calculated determinations, certain kinds of treatments in certain kinds of situations will be a priori excluded as too costly, too futile, or too inequitable based on limited resources. Second, all intra-system medical decisions for or against treatment must be centered on the patient's best interests, (for the most part) narrowly conceived. We can stretch this concept "not only to include familial burden, but one's social responsibilities," but this is only acceptable for those without a good prognosis — that is, "given a *severely* retarded, intractably pained, or permanently non-conscious infant" (309, emphasis added). In such cases, "social burden acts as a corroborating, possibly balance-tipping factor in determining patient well-being, but never as a lone criterion placed over and against the total best interests of the non-competent handicapped newborn" (324).

## Sparks: Critique

Sparks is largely onboard with the basic direction of this book. He simply has a worry (shared by many previously considered authors, though in a less narrow context) that considering social factors in the benefit/burden calculation at the micro/clinical level has dangers (both theoretical and practical) that make it prohibitive. Recall that he admits that Catholic teaching on ordinary and extraordinary means "ushered in the possibility of expanding the notion of the patient-person and of his/her best interests to include such social components as cost and burden to affected others, but always as *subsidiary elements* of the patient's interests, holistically considered, never as distinctive counter-claims" (emphasis added). But this way of thinking about the patient's interests could benefit from a critique offered in light of the moral anthropology offered by Catholic social teaching. The just claims that others in society have on us are not "counter" to or "distinctive" from what is in our best interest. In fact, there *are no interests* of our own that should not always and directly be evaluated in light of the claims of others. The idea that social components such as cost and burden to affected others are "subsidiary" elements of a patient's interest misses the central point of Catholic moral anthropology outlined above. If physicians have a duty to respect the "total best interests" of their patients, they must do so in light of empirical and theological facts: this is impossible to evaluate except in terms of one's fundamental and intrinsic sociality — on the part of the physician and her patient, both of whom have social duties in play.[59] Thus, the distinction Sparks wishes to make between considering social factors as primary on the level of social policy and on the "bedside/cribside" level is a false one. In both cases, policy makers and clinicians are obligated to do what is in the best interests of the newborn, not from an individualistically narrow point of view, but from a truly "total best interests" point of view — which includes the just claims of others to our resources.

Sparks does seem to accept, at least in part, the idea that "one's social responsibilities" could be part of one's best interests. However, he allows for this to be considered only in situations where treatment is of the most seriously imperiled newborns. That is, situations in which treatment "may constitute too much burden for too little medical and experiential benefit." In such cases, social factors only compound "an already negative prognosis." But again, given the moral anthropology of Catholic social teaching, there is no reason to accept this narrow understanding. Indeed, *everyone* is enjoined to refrain from using resources in a way that is disproportionate with the common good. And if one takes seriously the idea that even the most imperiled newborns have the same moral status as an older or more healthy human person, then in limiting this duty to only the sickest newborns, Sparks seems to undercut his own goal of avoiding bias against those patients least able to assert their rights and needs in the decision-making debate. No, it does seem at least theoretically possible (we will get into the practical

---

59. To this point I have spoken in generalities about such a duty and how it would play out in an NICU. The final chapter of this book will deal with these practical and specific questions in some detail.

specifics in chapter 4) that even less seriously imperiled infants (or, for that matter, *any* imperiled patient) may have a duty to refuse or withdraw treatment that is disproportionate with the common good.

Recall also Sparks's worry about abuse and a slippery slope leading toward the denigration of the inherent personhood of the infant if, at the bedside or cribside level, we directly considered social factors as primary. He buttresses this claim by pointing out that we seldom force competent patients to adhere to duties of social responsibility when it comes to treatment decisions, and this is evidence that, in even making the argument, his opponent is already treating the imperiled newborn as less than a full person. Three responses can be given that go beyond the one offered in chapter 2 to a similar line of argument. First, one needs to reiterate the principle of Catholic social teaching that *everyone* is enjoined to refrain from using resources in a way that is disproportionate with the common good. Indeed, though it goes beyond the scope of this book, other kinds of treatments designed for competent adults (cosmetic surgery, certain procedures near the end of life, etc.) might also be disproportionate with the common good and ruled out on that basis. Second, given Sparks's methodological principles, why would not the same worry apply in the macro or policy level? Depending on what the policy is (nontreatment of all infants born under 500 grams, for instance), one might "denigrate the personhood" of many more human infants than if one left it to the clinician on a case-by-case basis. Third, one cannot properly evaluate the relative benefits/burdens of treatment — and therefore the socially aware best interests of the infant — by considering only general trends on a policy level. Many judgment calls will have to be made by clinicians on a case-by-case basis, and this will require these clinicians to evaluate the infant with regard to the social totality of her best interests.

Sparks is understandably worried that putting a clinician in this role might undermine patient dignity in an unacceptable way. After all, modern-day bioethics grew out of a World War II context in which Nazi physicians engaged in precisely this kind of activity. However, the idea of physicians taking into account social factors in a primary way is not as radical as Sparks makes it seem. Joseph Fins argues that cost-cutting measures taken by hospitals and clinics mean that "physicians are no longer able to practice in economic isolation. As practitioners in economically strapped hospitals or in HMOs, physicians often encounter a conflict of interest between satisfying the patient needs and meeting their institution's demands."[60] And while it is true that the American Medical Association Code of Ethics explicitly demands that the physician act solely as a patient advocate, interestingly, it also notes that "Physicians as citizens have a responsibility to participate and to contribute their professional expertise in decisions made at the societal level regarding the allocation of health resources."[61] They make the very strong claim that a physician who acts clinically without considering costs and then politically advocates cost containment becomes a victim of an "untenable hypocrisy."

Cost containment is not the only situation in which physicians do not give a treatment that is disproportionate with the common good. Take the decision whether or not to prescribe an antibiotic. Fins rightly points out that although "an individual patient might conceivably benefit from a more powerful antibiotic that might marginally improve therapy, the use of the fail-safe drug is limited to well circumscribed situations by the broader needs of the community."[62] The physician weighs the benefit of giving the drug to the individual against the harm of increased drug-resistance within a given population. If the treatment is disproportionate with the common good, then the physician often will not prescribe the drug — even though it may well benefit the patient. No, the idea that Sparks is attacking is not so radical after all and certainly does not violate the goods of medicine or the time-honored relationship between physicians and patients.

What, then, are we to make of the part of Sparks's second methodological claim in which he says social burden on others should act only as a "corroborating, possibly balance-tipping factor" in treatment decisions by clinicians? While the fundamental sociality, and therefore

---

60. Joseph J. Fins, "The Rationing of Health Care: A Doctor's Dilemma," *Journal of Religion and Health* 32, no. 1 (Spring 1993): 13.

61. Quoted in Fins, "Rationing of Health Care," 14. Without a moral anthropology that is cut out of the same cloth as that of Catholic social teaching, it looks like the AMA Code of Ethics has a contradiction here — for if one considers the patient's interests from a narrow point of view, it seems obvious that these will directly conflict with those of the institution in many situations. That the code includes both is interesting because, if it is not seen as a contradiction, it is an implicit acceptance of Catholic social teaching — like anthropology.

62. Fins, "Rationing of Health Care," 14.

social duties, of the human person has already called this kind of reasoning into serious question, the absolutely overwhelming social consequences in play make one wonder if such a narrow understanding is commensurate with the seriousness of the social situation. Consider how Mary J. McDonough nicely summarizes the health care situation in the United States as this book goes to press:[63]

> Today the healthcare system in the United States is a mire of rapidly increasing costs and continually declining of insured. Efforts to achieve universal healthcare coverage have chronically failed. Yet healthcare costs are rapidly rising. In 1970, 7.6 percent of the nation's gross domestic product (GDP) was spent on healthcare. By 2004, that figure had risen to 15 percent, the highest in the world. Moreover, 2003 insurance premiums rose 13.9 percent, greatly outpacing the 2.2 percent inflation rate. That was the third consecutive year of double-digit premium increases and represented the greatest increase since 1990. The number of uninsured people is growing as well. In 2004 approximately 44.5 million people in the United States were uninsured. There is a general agreement on why affordable, fair distribution of healthcare is growing increasingly difficult: the rising number of elderly people as a significant proportion of the population, the impact of new technologies and the intensified use of older ones, and an increasing public demand for better healthcare.[64]

To get a sense of the kind of numbers we are talking about, consider that 15 percent of the 2004 GDP is approximately $1,647,000,000,000.

Neonatal intensive care is already "one of the highest single hospital costs — more than 25% of the country's entire maternal-newborn budget," and this cost shows no sign of doing anything other than growing. "The number of neonatologists has doubled since 1985,"[65] and profitability and cost of NICU treatments, length of NICU stays,

---

63. Again, the need to consciously ration health care resources only becomes more explicit in the happy scenario where many of these millions become covered by Medicaid.

64. Mary Joan McDonough, *Can a Health Care Market Be Moral? A Catholic Vision* (Washington, D.C.: Georgetown University Press, 2007), 2-3.

65. Peter A. Clark, *To Treat or Not to Treat: The Ethical Methodology of Richard A. McCormick, S.J., as Applied to Treatment Decisions for Handicapped Newborns* (Omaha: Creighton University Press, 2003), 24.

and new NICUs built continue to grow dramatically.[66] These considerations, dramatic as they are, constitute only a fraction of the total cost
of the treatment of imperiled newborns. As Sparks himself notes, the
"initial neonatal costs are multiplied many times over if one takes into
account the expense of long term care — repeated surgeries, hospitalization, therapy, special education, family support services, and possible institutionalization."[67] These costs are even more dramatic when
one considers the rapid rise of health care costs over the lifetime of the
patient.

  The dramatic numbers involved in the cost of health care resources,
and those affected by their distribution, are certainly added reasons to
reject Sparks's claim that social burden should be a mere "balance-
tipping" factor in NICU treatment decisions. This becomes even more
convincing when one considers that "society bears the brunt of these expenses in terms of Medicaid and insurance payments as well as the cost
of maintaining institutional facilities."[68] One can see this most clearly if
one looks at how Medicaid is impacted. Though much more will be said
about the specifics in the following chapter (and much depends on
what socioeconomic clientele the unit serves), because a clear majority
of NICU infants are funded mostly by Medicaid, decisions about treatment directly affect others whose health care resources come from the
same Medicaid pool. In a very real way, then, decisions about Medicaid
treatment (on both the policy and the clinical levels) are analogous to
decisions made in a battlefield triage situation (on the levels of both
policy and decisions by the medic). In both situations the relevant resources (money spent on a patient versus time spent on a patient) are
limited such that difficult and tragic decisions need to be made — for
some are going to get inadequate care and are going to die. Decisions
not to treat patients that might have survived, on the basis of due proportion with the common good, do not violate the good of medicine on
the battlefield or in the disaster area and, this book argues, do not violate the good of medicine in the NICU. Indeed, it upholds the duty of
medicine to treat the best interests of the patient in the way that is most

  66. John D. Lantos and William Meadow, *Neonatal Bioethics: The Moral Challenges of
Medical Innovation* (Baltimore: Johns Hopkins University Press, 2006), 177, 130-35.
  67. Sparks, *To Treat,* 230.
  68. Sparks, *To Treat,* 230.

authentically aware of the true dignity, best interests, and quality of life of the human person. However, the claimed analogy between a battle-field triage situation and Medicaid treatment[69] is controversial and warrants a more detailed underpinning.

## Medicaid and Triage

Medicaid is the largest public health insurance program in the United States and provides assistance to more than 50 million Americans at the cost of over $300 billion.[70] Medicaid programs are currently administered and partially funded by individual states, but the federal government provides significant support with the requirement that states fully cover low-income children and some pregnant women — after which they can use monies to cover other people.[71] To see the analogy between Medicaid and a triage situation, it is instructive to examine a particular state-run Medicaid program, in this case Tennessee.[72] The

69. The analogy between battlefield triage and NICU treatment decisions works best when applied to a person or entity who has a special concern for the common good — just as a battlefield medic must consider the common good of all her soldier-patients. This means that the analogy works less well when it involves a parent making a decision for his newborn because of the special concern a parent must and should have for his child.

70. Some might wonder, especially in a book written in sympathy with Catholic social teaching, if Medicaid is a good choice for comparison here. If one claims to have a preferential option for the poor, a central principle of CST, how could one be willing to dramatically limit neonatal care for the (largely) impoverished people who qualify for Medicaid? This is an important question — but it must be seen in the context of the full constructive proposal argued for in the final chapter. Here are two preliminary suggestions: first, when changes are made to Medicaid, the private insurance companies almost always follow suit — which means that changes to Medicaid will likely trickle down to the rest of the population; second, those who are responsible for making decisions about how Medicaid funds are distributed should do so without reference to factors over which they have no control — like how well their program is funded in relationship to other programs. Their primary concern should be with regard to the things over which they *do* have control: just and proportional allocation of resources within the Medicaid population.

71. "Medicaid Squeeze," *Online Newshour,* March 2, 2005; http://www.pbs.org/newshour/bb/health/jan-june05/medicaid_3-02.html (accessed October 16, 2007).

72. All material on the program taken from Families USA, "Unwilling Volunteers:

state's Medicaid program, TennCare, was once considered a model for the country. In 1994, the program was financially sound and had helped to drop Tennessee's uninsured level to one of the lowest in the country. But TennCare ran into problems in 1999 due to several factors: poor management, underfunding, and, perhaps most importantly, dramatically rising costs due to medical inflation. Either unable or unwilling to secure more funding, TennCare was forced to drop approximately 120,000 people from the program beginning in August 2005. And those who remained in the program were subject to one of the strictest prescription drug limits anywhere in the country: adults could get only five drug prescriptions filled per month — three generics and two brand-name drugs. No safety net was in place for those who were dropped altogether. Eighteen months after the cuts began, the state launched a program to help the "uninsurable" — people lucky enough to have had access to private insurance but who had since been rejected. Such programs were too little too late and served only a fraction of those who had been dropped from TennCare.

The best way to understand the dramatic effect this had on the lives of real people[73] is to hear their stories — especially in light of the fact that they are almost never told, while stories about newborns make sexy headlines.

- *Jerry Springfield* (Jackson). Jerry has muscle spasms in his heart — a condition that requires him to take eight pills every day and to see a cardiologist. He has no income other than $157 per month in food stamps, and he lives with his parents. After he was dropped from TennCare, he showed up for a cardiologist appointment and was told that his insurance would no longer pay for visits. "I couldn't pay for the appointment without TennCare coverage," Jerry said, "so I simply didn't see my doctor that day." Even with his discount card, his drugs cost $400 — which he cannot afford. Recently, he has experienced severe pain in his right arm that prevents him from raising it. "I would have liked to go to the doctor for it, but I couldn't afford

---

Tennesseans Forced Out of Health Care"; http://www.familiesusa.org/resources/ publications/reports/tenncare-report.html (accessed October 16, 2007).

73. Knowing the personal stories of those affected will be important later in responding to some anti-triage-analogy arguments.

to," he said. Jerry has tried to get on disability insurance, but his application was denied.

- *Janice Harris* (Nashville). Janice used to work on a regular basis, but after a car accident left her with a severe back injury (requiring four surgeries), she was unable to work — and when she was denied disability her income dropped to zero. The offender in the car accident paid medical bills related to the accident, but her other medical and psychological ailments were not covered: kidney stones, esophagus stretching, and clinical depression. Losing TennCare has forced her into severe indignities and even life-threatening situations. When her esophagus gets inflamed, she has no money to treat it — thus, when it gets bad, "all I can eat is baby food." She has also been unable to see a doctor about a lump in her breast even though she has a family history of breast cancer.

- *Aaron England* (Crossville). Aaron worked for twenty-three years, never had health insurance, and luckily has led a healthy life. However, this caught up with him all at once when he developed a triple hernia, a serious and chronic infection, and a cancerous thyroid. Though he originally qualified for TennCare, in the midst of the treatment of these problems, he was removed. He has been surviving because of the free drug samples he gets from his doctor, but he can no longer afford to get his blood drained of excess cells from his infection, so he is at growing risk of having a stroke. Asked what he would tell the governor about the TennCare cuts, he said, "I would say that he is going to kill a lot of innocent people. Believe it or not, there are a lot of people worse off than I am."

These tragedies are totally unacceptable given the resources of the country in which these patients live — and one solution to these problems, certainly, would have been to better fund TennCare such that needy people like these would not have been dropped.[74] However, when one views Medicaid programs in isolation from this unfortunate and unjust underfunding (as one would have to do when making public policy about allocation of Medicaid funds or clinical treatment decisions for those on Medicaid), one can see how very much like a triage situation it is. Because a Medicaid program has limited resources, and

74. These kinds of considerations will be taken up in the conclusion of the book.

because the medical need in virtually every state dramatically outpaces the capacity of these resources, decisions to spend resources in a particular way necessitate that certain needy others will not get the resources they need — regardless of how the money is allocated. As we see with TennCare, tragically, this means that some people will die who otherwise would have survived.[75]

This is precisely the case in a typical triage situation on the battlefield, in a disaster area, or in a hospital — except that the social resource in question is not money but time. Consider the classical triage classifications and priority codes:

>"**Emergent**" (or "**Red**"). Priority 1 is given to critically ill patients who may survive with intervention that does not consume significant resources and personnel, that is, patients who need immediate surgery to save life or limb, using minimal operation time, and who are expected to have a good quality of survival.
>
>"**Urgent**" (or "**Yellow**"). Priority 2 is given to patients who are likely to survive and remain stable for several hours by means of stabilization, that is, patients who need time-consuming surgery and whose lives will not be jeopardized by delay.
>
>"**Nonurgent**" (or "**Green**"). Priority 3 is given to patients who have minor injuries that may be treated by those with minimal training, that is, patients who can wait until other injured patients have been cared for.
>
>"**Expectant**" (or "**Black**"). No obvious priority. Patients who have overwhelming injuries with little chance for survival and patients with severe injuries who are not expected to survive unless time-consuming care is almost immediate. The only priority is palliative care and comfort measures to those dying.[76]

The key to triage is to apportion the available resources in connection with the common good of the entire community under consideration of the triage physician. The good aimed at might be different de-

---

75. Indeed, the Urban Institute and the Institute for Medical Analysis estimate that many thousands in the United States die from preventable disease simply because they are uninsured; see http://www.urban.org/UploadedPDF/411588_uninsured_dying.pdf (accessed August 6, 2008).

76. Mikko A. Salo, "Triage in Social Policy," *Acta Philosophica Fennica* 68 (2001): 156.

pending on the circumstances,[77] but most often the goal is to save as many lives as possible. For, as John Kilner points out, the right to life is not a claim to equal resources — rather, the "real claim of each person . . . is that his life be valued equally with all others — which in turn necessitates that two rather than one be selected"[78] in a case where either one or two persons in a group of three could be saved. Though it is difficult and tragic to admit, patients "with a black card are thought to need too many resources which would deprive more viable patients and who, therefore, may have to be allocated low priority due to limited resources."[79] The variables of number of patients, the severity of the injuries, and the amount of medical resources all help to determine who gets what kind of priority. If the number of patients is high and the injuries life-threatening, "the only care that may take place is in the form of rapid life-saving manoeuvres. When resources are limited — and they nearly always are — in these situations, many patients who might normally receive maximum medical treatment are left to die at the scene because they will consume too much time and resources better allocated to others who have a better chance of surviving."[80]

Calling this "triage reasoning" (or a similar phrase) calls to mind an exceptional or uncommon case, and therefore it might seem that such reasoning applies only to exceptional and uncommon cases like the battlefield or a disaster area. However, as Kilner makes clear, this kind of reasoning applies in any situation where there are "disproportionate resources." Take the very generic situation in which three people are equally in need of certain scarce lifesaving resources. One requires the entire amount available, whereas the other two each require only half. In such a case, all else being equal, "it is right to save the two rather than risking likelihood that only one would be saved."[81] What

77. For instance, in a particular battlefield situation one might use "reverse triage," in which soldiers who through medical intervention could be ready to fight again relatively soon might receive first priority whereas those who could benefit from treatment but who will not fight again (leg amputees, for instance) will receive less priority despite having a more severe injury.

78. John F. Kilner, "A Moral Allocation of Scarce Lifesaving Medical Resources," *Journal of Religious Ethics* 9, no. 2 (Fall 1981): 264.

79. Salo, "Triage in Social Policy," 156.

80. Salo, "Triage in Social Policy," 156.

81. Kilner, "A Moral Allocation," 263.

this means, then, is that far from limiting this kind of reasoning to exceptional situations, we should broaden it out to any situation in which we are dealing with these three conditions:

a patient population,

a significant portion of that population in need of lifesaving therapies, and

limited medical resources such that, regardless of how we use them, some patients will die who otherwise could have been saved.

If these three conditions are met, then we should use something like triage reasoning in determining how to allocate our medical resources. Just as a battlefield or disaster-area medic would not randomly allocate resources by a lottery, or according to the first patient that met her gaze, or by what a market determined, neither should any of those factors determine how to allocate the medical resources present in public health programs like Medicaid or any other program that meets the three criteria above. Instead, all physicians — whether in a disaster area, an NICU, or a battlefield — should always be allocating resources with the patient's total best interests in mind; if I am correct, this includes avoiding treatments that are disproportionate with the common good.

In May 1990, the state of Oregon attempted to do precisely this with their Medicaid system.[82] Much more will be said about this in chapter 4; here we want to get a glimpse of how this kind of triage reasoning might work in practice. The high cost of health care was making it impossible for Oregon to cover all its poor who had severe medical problems. So they created a list of over 1,600 diseases, disorders, and conditions and ranked them according to which had the most favorable cost-of-treatment to benefit-of-treatment ratio. At some place on the list, to be determined by the amount of money available to the Medicaid program, a cutoff would be imposed and Medicaid would refuse to pay for treatment of the conditions below the cutoff. This was the trade-off for getting all those below the poverty level covered under Oregon Medicaid.

82. Robert McCarthy, "Triage for the Poor in Oregon — Recasting of Medicaid Payment Disorder Ranking," *Business and Health* (April 1991).

However, the algorithm programmed into a computer to determine the list (which did consider factors like life expectancy and quality of life) put headache and thumb sucking higher on the list than life-threatening diseases such as viral pneumonia and cystic fibrosis. Subsequently, an eleven-member panel called the Oregon Health Commission (five physicians, one social worker, one nurse, and four representatives from patient-advocacy groups) completely recast the list in light of some different human judgments and values. Esoteric diseases were put toward the bottom of the list, and life-threatening conditions and preventive care were given much higher priority. Not surprisingly, however, some life-threatening conditions and diseases ended up below the line. The new list bottomed out with AIDS — given that the survival rate was less than 10 percent over five years. Interestingly, especially for chapter 4 of this book, maternity and healthy-baby care ranked very high, but treatment of extremely low-birth-weight babies (less than 1.1 pounds, or about 500 grams), though they were able to be saved in some cases, was ranked rather low.[83]

It seems clear that in any situation in which the above three criteria are met, regardless of how the resources are distributed, people are going to die. The reasoning of the advocates of the Oregon Medicaid plan, and of this book, is that people are already dying as an indirect result of how we allocate resources — but in a largely unregulated, unsystematic, and definitely unjust way. This is a tragic and avoidable situation. But seen through the lens of those who have no control over the amount of resources at the disposal of programs like Medicaid, and yet still have to make resource-allocation and treatment decisions, how much better to make choices systematically in proportion with the common good of one's patient population?

83. As we will see in chapter 4, having a blanket criterion like gram weight is not enough when coming up with NICU policies that respect treatments only insofar as they are in due proportion with the common good. Sparks could be happy with something like the Oregon plan because it is on the macro or policy level (though it is still unclear how it denigrates, say, AIDS patients any less than if the decision not to treat was made at the micro level), but he could not accept what will be required of the neonatologist insofar as she is forced to make a determination "at the cribside."

## Medicaid and Triage: Some Understandable Concerns

Many object to using triage as an analogy for Medicaid — or as an analogy for any kind of medical program. And they have convincing reasons for doing so. One who makes a particularly strong case is Benjamin Freedman. Though his main worry is that we preference the treatment of the sick over preventive care of the healthy, he gives us several reasons to be skeptical of the triage analogy.[84] He grants the truth of the claim that something like triage medicine yields the best "return on the dollar" — but only if one accepts that return being concerned with producing "better mortality and morbidity rates."[85] Freedman suggests that this kind of return on the dollar should not be our number one priority. He reviews the arguments of several thinkers who have written on allocation of scarce resources who agree "on just this principle: that man should be prevented from deciding the fate of men."[86] He quotes Paul Ramsey, who claims that in allocation of sparse medical resources among equally needy persons, "an extension of God's indiscriminate care into human affairs requires random selection and forbids godlike judgments that one man is worth more than another."[87] We should not be prepared to adopt a policy, Freedman argues, that will make it apparent that the claims of lives in dire need can be adjudicated by human beings. This is precisely what the triage analogy asks us to do.

Another argument Freedman convincingly uses against the claim that "we should save as many lives as we can" invokes a significant distinction between mere statistics and the worth of a known, individual life. In fact, he claims this is how we already do things, uncontroversially, in other contexts. Consider that "society seems to have taken advantage of the psychosymbolic advantage of showing commitment to the dignity and worth of the individual life (while neglecting, sometimes woefully, the good of the 'faceless statistic')."[88] Indeed, we man-

84. Benjamin Freedman, "Case for Medical Care, Inefficient or Not," *Hastings Center Report* 7, no. 2 (April 1977): 31-39.

85. Freedman, "Case for Medical Care," 31.

86. Freedman, "Case for Medical Care," 33.

87. Paul Ramsey, *The Patient as Person: Explorations in Medical Ethics,* Lyman Beecher Lectures at Yale University (New Haven: Yale University Press, 1970), 259.

88. Freedman, "Case for Medical Care," 34.

date the use of only relatively cheap and therefore relatively limited safety features on our cars, etc., even though we know that, statistically, more people will die than if we had mandated more expensive and better features. However, in contrast, we spare no expense to save the coal mine disaster victim. What is going on here? Freedman suggests that we have a (good and healthy) bias in favor of attention of the individual over and against the mere statistic. For, it appears, "No one seems to be making the decisions to take human lives and, therefore, no blatant infringement of the commitment to human life as sacred occurs."[89] In a triage-like situation, by contrast, a human person is directly choosing not to save a particular life, in favor of another life or lives, and this infringes on human dignity. It is a problem inherent in "dealing with statistics, with large numbers of people as an undifferentiated mass, thus excluding individuation of treatment."[90] Rather, we should err on the side of policy that supports "freedom and individualism" rather than the "opposite" that a more statistics-based approach produces.

James Burtchaell also communicates some convincing worries about the triage analogy.[91] To begin with, even if triage reasoning seems justified, "it has a way of consuming a person. For a doctor, the fibers of whose self are braided into lifelines of generous concern, it snarls the soul, not simply to lose a patient to death, but to mark him or her for death. It may require uncommonly high and durable virtue to perform this task without making a vice out of a necessity" (506). This worry is magnified in that triage seems to be too easily invoked in ethical reasoning. For "in a world where medical resources are never likely to satisfy medical needs, is not every day one of triage?" (507). Do we really want all physicians who deal with life-threatening illnesses to "snarl their soul" in calculating the relative value of their patients?

Burtchaell acknowledges that if we "grant the battle exists," then triage and battlefield reasoning seems to be a kind of necessary evil. But he asks, "Why grant the battle in the first place?" Why participate in the evil structures that force us into such tragically person-

---

89. Freedman, "Case for Medical Care," 34.
90. Freedman, "Case for Medical Care," 443.
91. James Burtchaell, "How Much Should a Child Cost? A Response to Paul Johnson," in *On Moral Medicine*, 503-11. In-text page numbers in the remainder of this section refer to Burtchaell's article.

consuming situations? He cites an example of a Nazi program once proposed to Adolf Eichmann: "There is an imminent danger that not all the Jews can be supplied with food in the coming winter. We must seriously consider if it would not be more humane to finish off the Jews, insofar as they are not fit for labor mobilization, with some quick-acting means. In any case this would be more agreeable than to let them die of hunger" (507). There is no triage, Burtchaell argues, when the same people who offer the most humane or just solution in a tragic situation are themselves participating in — or even the direct cause of — the social structures that forced the tragedy in the first place.

Burtchaell concludes with the by now familiar slippery slope argument — or what he calls "the possibility of great mischief." He is worried that any kind of shift away from a physician focusing on the (narrowly considered) best interests of the patient in front of him will lead us down a path we do not want to take. He again cites a Nazi example in support of his claim. In attempting to get the Dutch physicians onboard with what German doctors were doing, they were not told to "send your chronic patients to death factories" or that you "must give lethal injections at Government request in your offices." Rather, the Reich commissioner of the Netherlands territories gave the following order: "It is the duty of the doctor, through advice and effort, conscientiously and to the best of his ability, to assist as helper the person entrusted to his care in the maintenance, improvement and re-establishment of his vitality, physical efficiency and health. The accomplishment of this duty is a public task" (507). The Dutch physicians unanimously rejected the order, because they knew the slippery slope down which it would lead — "namely, the concentration of their efforts on mere rehabilitation of the sick for useful labor, and the abolition of medical secrecy" (507). It is the first, slight step away from an essential principle that is the most important one. Because they did not step away from their principles, "not a single euthanasia or non-therapeutic sterilization was recommended or participated in by any Dutch physician" (508).

So while Catholic teaching on ordinary/extraordinary means is correct that death is not the ultimate enemy, "perhaps abandonment is" (508). Triage-like reasoning forces us to abandon patients on some level — so what is left to stop this reasoning from mushrooming out to other, less comfortable, levels? This, after all, is what happened in Nazi

Germany and was only avoided by the Dutch physicians when they refused to take even one step down that road. If we use a kind of reasoning that demands that we abandon patients within Medicaid, and then specifically for imperiled newborns within Medicaid, will we really be able to hang on to the truth that "that stunted, afflicted fellow human of [ours] is already as invaluably valuable as he or she ever will or would be" (508)? Or will we slide down the slippery slope to something that no one advocating the first step ever intended?

## A Response to the Concerns

Both Freedman and Burtchaell make powerful arguments — worthy of a considered and careful response. What of Freedman's claim that "men should not be deciding the fate of men"? That, in a case of limited resources, we should imitate God's "indiscriminate" giving of resources and randomly select those who get them? There are at least two important responses to this move. First, we should remind ourselves that *it is already the case that human beings are deciding the fate of other human beings.* All one need do is look at Medicaid in Tennessee or Oregon or any number of other states to realize that nonrandom choices are being made as to who is "in" and who is "out" when it comes to who receives the limited number of community resources. The primary argument of this book is not that we should use Catholic social teaching as a guide for deciding the fate of other human beings rather than using a random method; the argument is that we should use Catholic social teaching as a guide for deciding the fate of other human beings rather than the current methods: market-driven decisions, bias in favor of the politically powerful or sympathetic, etc.[92]

But perhaps this response would not be satisfying to Freedman — he could grant that a method based on Catholic social teaching is better than what we are currently doing, but it is still not the ideal. Again, we should imitate God rather than human beings — and humbly submit to a truly random distribution. However, if one takes the principles of Catholic social teaching seriously, this simply will not do.

---

92. Much more will be said about how these methods work in practice in the first part of chapter 4.

For God, from the perspective of this tradition, is certainly *not* indiscriminate in giving attention and concern for humanity. Catholic social teaching has articulated this as a "preferential option for the poor." Pope Leo XIII said, "When it comes to protecting the rights of individuals, the poor and the helpless have a claim to special consideration."[93] John Paul II also invokes "the option or love of preference for the poor. This is an option, or a special form of primacy in the exercise of Christian charity, to which the whole tradition of the Church bears witness. It affects the life of each Christian inasmuch as he or she seeks to imitate the life of Christ, but it applies equally to our social responsibilities and hence to our manner of living, and to the logical decisions to be made concerning the ownership and use of goods."[94] Charles Curran notes that we normally think, especially in the West, of preference or bias as a negative thing. However, this is not what our faith teaches us. Our God has a bias in favor of the poor and the lowly. And it is precisely this bias that strengthens the common good of all.[95] Those poor who are unjustly being dropped from Medicaid have a special claim to our attention — and cannot be dismissed in a random distribution process.

Recall also that Freedman refers to the "faceless statistic" in almost disparaging terms. A "statistics-based" approach like triage puts more value on "undifferentiated mass" than on the individual dignity of the person right in front of you. Indeed, we as a culture do seem to care more about making automobiles affordable than about the "faceless statistics" that would be saved by making them safer and more expensive. If Freedman's point here is simply about what *is* the case, rather than about what *should* be the case, then he certainly has a strong argument. It surely is the case that when someone is a "faceless statistic," that person's dignity often comes second to the dignity of others who are "known" to the person making choices that affect them all. But from the point of view of Catholic social teaching — which claims that "all really are responsible for all" and that we should have a preferential option for the poor — this is definitely not a good thing. Recall Catho-

93. Leo XIII, *Rerum Novarum* (New York: Paulist, 1900), 29.

94. John Paul II, *Sollicitudo Rei Socialis,* 42.

95. Charles E. Curran, *Catholic Social Teaching, 1891-Present: A Historical, Theological, and Ethical Analysis,* Moral Traditions Series (Washington, D.C.: Georgetown University Press, 2002), 173-214.

lic social teaching's insight about the "multiplied ties" of human persons in today's globalized world — and Whitmore's insistence that this means we are all part of a *world* community. It follows from this that our social responsibilities go well beyond those that are "known" to us; rather, the so-called faceless statistic is a human person toward whom we have a strong social duty as fellow members of a world community. Pope Benedict reminds us of this in his introduction to his latest encyclical when he claims that any effort to obtain the common good "cannot fail to assume the dimensions of the whole human family, that is to say, the communities of peoples and nations."[96]

Indeed, Freedman's argument helps remind us that part of this duty includes making the "undifferentiated mass" of needy poor *known* to us and others so that more will be moved to engage their social duties toward them. This is precisely why it is so important to tell the stories of people like those who were kicked out of Medicaid — they cease to become faceless statistics and get closer to becoming our sisters and brothers calling out for our aid.[97] But whatever the case about their relative levels of familiarity, the poor should still be the focus for our duties as members of a world community.

Let us move to Burtchaell's claims. Recall that he allows for triage reasoning "if we grant the battle" — and then calls into question doing precisely that. But say we accept this move — how would it play out practically for a battlefield or disaster-area medic? Let us suppose that the medic comes across the first wounded person and determines that this life could be saved, but it will take her undivided attention for the next hour. Let us also suppose that, based on her previous experience and training, she determines that she could instead use the time to save at least five other people who otherwise would die. If she chooses to save the first person she comes across, what should she say in response to the parents of the other wounded persons who died because she

96. Benedict XVI, *Caritas in Veritate*, 7.

97. Perhaps this kind of reasoning is also an indictment of what Freedman also notes "is the case" — the preference of cheaper automobiles over saving the lives of faceless statistics. If we were made aware of the mangled bodies that resulted from these choices, and the wailing of their friends and family members that followed, perhaps we would take a different approach. Whether or not the lives actually are more than faceless statistics to us, however, is not the point. All human beings are part of one world community — and we have social duties toward all.

chose to help the first person? That she "refuses to grant the battle"? Aside from the inappropriateness of this answer with reference to disaster-area (perhaps after a hurricane or some such event where there is no military battle), it is wholly unsatisfactory with regard to justice considerations. The parents of those who died could rightly complain that the medic spent resources on one patient in a way that was disproportionate with the common good of the patient population of which their daughter or son was a part. There will always be mitigating factors that make a particular treatment decision more or less difficult, but one should never retreat from one's duty to the common good simply because the circumstances force one into a difficult situation.

But perhaps Burtchaell could make a version of the common good argument here. Like many others, he invokes the "slippery slope" of any reasoning that forces us to abandon a patient. With this worry in mind, perhaps he could argue that a treatment that is disproportionate with the common good is in fact the one that opens the door to other more serious kinds of patient abandonment: something like what happened in Nazi Germany, for instance. Surely the risk of that kind of thing happening is a more serious threat to the common good than the alternative. But the response to Burtchaell here must be, again, that *patients are already being abandoned either way*. If the medic "refuses to grant the battle" and stops to help the first patient for an hour, then she has abandoned the other patients — even though they might be over the next hill and she never has to look them in the face. The same is true within a given Medicaid population. If we "refuse to grant the battle," then we leave market, political, and other forces to abandon patients — like those from TennCare described above. The question is what *kind* of abandonment are we going to practice?[98] Are we simply going to ignore the wounded soldiers over the hill and tend to the person in front of us? Or, coming upon the first soldier, will we give him a loving smile, a shot of morphine, briefly hold his hand, and then move on to another

---

98. This is true at least in the first stage of this battle for justice in health care. Admittedly, it does appear to be wrong and dangerous to be content with a situation that forces us to abandon patients in this way — especially given the resources that exist in our society. Though this book limits itself to arguments within our current system, the conclusion to this book makes explicit the idea that our current structure is not ideal and ought to be dramatically changed. Even the health care reform plans being proposed and debated as this book goes to press will leave many millions uninsured.

patient whose treatment would not be disproportionate with the common good?

But is not this last move horribly difficult? It is one thing to abandon someone that one never meets, but how could one look into the eyes of a dying patient, someone that could be saved, and then leave the patient to die? Would not repeated instances of this, as Burtchaell says, "snarl one's soul" and ultimately consume the humanity of anyone who practiced it? No doubt it would take the virtue of fortitude to undertake these kinds of difficult decisions, but fortitude is something that good physicians who deal with life-and-death issues possess in abundance already. How strong must one be to be called from a family holiday gathering to do hours of emergency surgery? How strong must one be to abandon the lifesaving treatment of a patient who has determined that further interventions are too burdensome? How strong must one be to break the news to a pregnant woman that she has uterine cancer? In addition, Fins reminds us that the kind of explicit rationing that goes on in triage situations "might be a less bitter pill" to swallow than the elixir of being forced to allocate resources based on a politics- and market-driven method. (Indeed, how strong must one be — how snarled one's soul — in accepting that one's choices are contributing to *that* utterly tragic state of affairs?) Accepting "at the outset that our resources for healthcare are limited" provides the proper context for use of those resources in a systematic manner.[99] The constraints imposed by the social quality of life model "may ultimately lead to improved medical care" by forcing us to examine critically our use of resources — and thus it would be far more likely to be "moral, logical, nonarbitrary and scientifically based."[100] Allocating scarce resources is not the first challenge to the dialectical relationship of medicine's obligations with a patient's expectations — nor will it be the last. However, by "acknowledging the true breadth of responsibility to the individual and to society, physicians could instill into the relationship a greater sense of community. This added dimension could deepen and define the fiduciary obligation and secure the relationship that binds us."[101]

99. Fins, "Rationing of Health Care," 15.
100. Fins, "Rationing of Health Care," 16.
101. Fins, "Rationing of Health Care," 18.

# CHAPTER 4

# A Constructive Proposal for Reforming the Treatment and Care of Imperiled Newborns

> *There is now much broader public awareness of the need for difficult choices to be made by the providers of national healthcare. We have discussed the difficult economic issues which have to be managed in neonatal medicine because more babies are able to survive than in the past. . . . Consequently, this has caused questioning of whether funds spent on resuscitating or prolonging the life of babies where the prognosis is very poor are spent appropriately.*
>
> Nuffield Council on Bioethics[1]

We have discussed three general approaches to the social quality of life model: one that supports a strong version of the model, one that rejects the model, and a third that supports a weak version of the model. Each has been found to be inadequate — and most obviously with regard to their understandings of the human person. It is difficult, however, to imagine another alternative: Are there logical pathways still open to us? The answer is yes, and the key is to remember the reason why the strong version of the model was rejected in chapter 1. Those who support a strong version almost always argue from the less-than-full personhood of the newborn. If the arguments of the preceding chapters are correct, one need not accept this understanding of the

---

1. Nuffield Council on Bioethics, "Critical Care Decisions in Fetal and Neonatal Medicine" (2006), 164.

moral status of infants to support a strong version of the social quality of life model. Indeed, when a military or disaster medic uses the strong version of this model for allocation of her resources, she is not making any claims about the moral status of those she chooses to treat and those she does not. In fact, it is presumed that each of her potential patients has the same moral status and therefore an equal right to her medical consideration. However, it does not follow from this moral status that all persons have a right to be treated, even if the treatment is necessary to preserve life and even if they are currently the patient "in front of" the physician, in a sense that is disproportionate with the common good. All one is entitled to is equal consideration with others in proportion with the common good of all. In tragic situations, this may mean that lifesaving treatment may be justifiably withheld from some persons.

But how should this play out *practically* for the subject of this book: the treatment and care of imperiled newborns? This is the central question of this final chapter. It will begin by exploring in some detail the facts of, and attitudes toward, treatment of such newborns in today's neonatal intensive care units (NICUs).[2] What kinds of outcomes can one expect based on a particular diagnosis? How reliable are such diagnoses? What sorts of economic considerations impact treatment in the NICU? The second part of the chapter will offer a critique of this current situation using a strong version of the social quality of life model in light of Catholic social teaching. It also will deal with a major objection that such a critique is best leveled at single-payer systems by raising the example of Medicaid, its relationship to the funding of NICU treatments, and how it serves as a favorable "test case" for the social quality of life model with respect to imperiled newborns. Perhaps the most prominent moral feature of certain NICU treatments funded by Medicaid is their disproportionality with other medical treatments funded by Medicaid. Having found the current situation wanting, and dramatically so, the chapter will make several suggestions for changing how resources are distributed in the NICU — first considering past models for rationing such as Oregon's "generic health states" list and

2. It will focus mainly on the United States, but practices from other developed countries (the U.K. and the Netherlands, for instance) will be brought in for the sake of comparison.

the "quality-adjusted life-year." Appropriating workable and attractive aspects from these models, the chapter will then make constructive proposals for the following: combating a general "culture of overtreatment" in the NICU, refusing to treat reliably diagnosed terminal cases, and rationing Medicaid NICU care. The chapter will offer and respond to several objections to the constructive proposals — including an internal critique based on the charge that the proposal is inconsistent with a preferential option for the poor.

## Basic Facts about Treatment of Imperiled Newborns in the NICU[3]

Before making a constructive proposal in applying the social quality of life model to the treatment of imperiled newborns, it is important to get a detailed picture of the facts, practices, and attitudes of the modern-day NICU. Neonatal treatment takes place within twenty-eight days of birth — infant mortality, however, "is defined as death before 1 year of age."[4] Three groups of babies are generally admitted to the NICU.

1. *Full-Term Babies with Acute Illnesses.* According to Lantos, these are usually the least ethically controversial cases as the problems that arise in decision making are similar to the problems of other high-risk patients at any age. These babies generally either get better quickly or die quickly, and the major ethical problems arise when treatment is only partially successful and the babies survive but with long-term complications from their acute illnesses.
2. *Babies with Congenital Anomalies.* These babies were the subject of many dramatic cases in the 1970s and 1980s — and in particular those born with syndromes like trisomy 21 and spina bifida. These cases are often complex, however, because the life-threatening disease or malformation is often something unrelated to the congeni-

---

3. The information in this section is taken from John D. Lantos and William Meadow, *Neonatal Bioethics: The Moral Challenges of Medical Innovation* (Baltimore: Johns Hopkins University Press, 2006).
4. Lantos and Meadow, *Neonatal Bioethics*, 13.

tal anomaly — for instance, a baby with trisomy 21 might also have an intestinal or cardiac malformation. In such cases the life can often be saved, but nothing can be done to treat the underlying anomaly; thus the choice is to either save a life full of significant impairment or let "nature take its course." The decision forces one to deal with difficult issues surrounding quality of life that go beyond mere medical indications for survival.[5]

3. *Babies with Extreme Prematurity.* These babies include all the considerations of the other two groups, but add another: long-term prognostic uncertainty. For any given baby, "the potential outcomes range from early death to late death to survival with severe, moderate, or mild disabilities, to survival with no long-term medical or neurodevelopmental problems. Furthermore, the disabilities associated with the 'disease' can be cognitive, pulmonary, intestinal, or cardiac or involve virtually any other organ system."[6] Since these babies will be a major focus of the social quality of life model in this book, much more will be said about this uncertainty later in the chapter.

Due in no small part to improvements in treating babies in the three groups above (along with improved nutrition and sanitation), infant mortality dropped dramatically in the twentieth century in the United States: from 55 in 1,000 in 1900 to 9 in 1,000 in 2000. More recently, *neonatal* mortality has plummeted from 19 per 1,000 in 1960 to 4 per 1,000 in 2000. However, Lantos argues that progress in improving birth-weight-specific rates of survival came to a halt in the mid-1990s. Breakthroughs in treatment like the use of surfactant and antenatal steroids came into regular use at this time, and it does not look as if there are new treatments on the horizon.[7]

5. The paradigmatic example here is that of Baby Doe in the 1980s. This was a pivotal case for a host of reasons — including a dramatic shift to a "culture of overtreatment" in the NICU that will be explored later in the chapter.

6. Lantos and Meadow, *Neonatal Bioethics,* 16.

7. Some work is being done on improving outcomes from respiratory failure (a major problem in extremely premature infants): liquid ventilation, high-frequency oscillatory ventilation, new drugs to treat underdeveloped lungs, and even the prospect of an artificial placenta that could be attached to the umbilical cord after birth. However, the lag time on research and development is so long (surfactant and antenatal steroids had

Though the innovation of neonatal care has brought about significant burdens — many of which are the subject of this book — there is no question that the benefits brought about have been absolutely remarkable. Before 1965, most of the babies weighing less than 1,500 grams at birth died. Today, more than 90 percent of them survive; a conservative estimate is that 20,000 infants per year now survive who otherwise would have died. Assuming a life expectancy of about eighty years, neonatal intensive care creates 1.6 million years of life — years that would have otherwise been lost — in the United States every year. In addition, studies have shown that one in eight births in the United States is premature — that number is growing and showing no sign of slowing down.[8] This means that the NICU will likely become even more important and add more life-years in the foreseeable future. Though from many perspectives this benefit is surely enough to overwhelm any burden, this book (and this chapter in particular) means to call such perspectives into serious question.

## Outcomes and Predictions[9]

Lantos goes so far as to argue that accurate predictions are "the basis for ethical decision making in the NICU."[10] For instance, if we can predict accurately that a particular treatment will be beneficial (the previous two chapters have attempted to show that what this means can be complex), it may be morally obligatory to continue or to initiate treatment — and if we know a treatment will fail it may be morally permitted (or even obligatory)[11] to refuse or discontinue treatment. The harder cases, of course, come when the predictions are not so certain —

---

clinical trials as early as the 1970s) that — for the foreseeable future at least — we will not have any new neonatal treatments.

8. See http://www.cnn.com/2008/HEALTH/conditions/06/20/premature.babies .ap/index.html (accessed June 20, 2008).

9. This section of the chapter will consider only short-term outcomes. Later in the chapter, and especially in response to a strong opposing argument that compares the costs of NICU care to other kinds of care, longer-term outcomes will be considered.

10. Lantos and Meadow, *Neonatal Bioethics,* 88.

11. One of the arguments this chapter will consider claims that some kinds of treatments are always wrong to administer.

in a kind of gray area of neonatal decision making. The gray area, described in terms of gestational age, is between twenty-two and twenty-six weeks; in weight it is between 500 and 850 grams. Below the low numbers almost no baby survives, and above the high numbers almost every baby lives. It stands to reason, then, not to treat babies below the low numbers and to treat the babies above the high numbers — but even if this is correct (and, all by itself, it may very well not be), what should be done in the gray area? The 1983 President's Commission on Bioethics suggested that parental preferences should determine treatment decisions.[12] However, clinical research over the last two decades has significantly narrowed the gray area (or at least made it less gray), such that (1) parents are now given much more accurate predictions with which to make ethical decisions, and (2) not all decisions by parents should be seen as having ethical defensibility in light of the data.

The most important factor to consider at birth, Lantos argues, is birth weight. In general, the heavier the baby, the better the chance of survival. However, another major factor to consider, more recent clinical research has found, is the "initial response" of the newborn child. Lantos found that, at least for the babies in the University of Chicago Hospital NICU (and this has been backed up by other studies), "more than half of the premature babies who ultimately died would die in the first three days of life, regardless of the treatment they received."[13] Prior to day four of postnatal life, the best predictor of outcomes is birth weight — but for babies who survive past this time, birth weight virtually disappears as a relevant predictor of survival. Indeed, the "600-gram babies who survive for three days do just as well as the 1000-gram babies who survive for three days." Not so long ago, it was presumed that the best time to make a decision about treatment was in the delivery room — and also that once a treatment decision was made it was largely irreversible. Lantos convincingly argues that this is not the case. Of all babies weighing 750 grams at birth, half will live and half will die, and it is impossible to tell from the gram weight alone

---

12. President's Commission for the Study of Ethical Problems in Medicine and Biomedical and Behavioral Research, *Deciding to Forego Life-Sustaining Treatment: A Report on the Ethical, Medical, and Legal Issues in Treatment Decisions* (Washington, D.C.: President's Commission for the Study of Ethical Problems in Medicine and Biomedical and Behavioral Research, 1983), 554.

13. Lantos and Meadow, *Neonatal Bioethics,* 90.

which will do what. Lantos argues that "One way to determine more accurately to which group a particular baby belongs is to treat all of the babies. The sickest babies then 'declare themselves' by dying in spite of medical treatment. The less sick babies also 'declare themselves' by improving over the first few days."[14]

But what to do after seventy-two hours? There are other predictive indicators to use at this point, but they are not well understood, need more study, and are very complex. One widely used metric is the SNAP (score for neonatal acute physiology) score, which incorporates thirty-seven physiological and biochemical markers: everything from heart rate to glucose level to oxygenation index. SNAP scores have been moderately helpful as predictors because they are significantly different for the babies who go on to die compared to those who go on to survive. However, SNAP has weaknesses too. One is that the scores are, again, most indicative of outcomes during the first three days of postnatal life. Later, "when the predictive value of birth weight decreases, and the SNAP score could potentially be a more clinically useful predictor, the differences between the SNAP scores of the two groups narrow."[15] Add to this the fact that (though its predictions of survival are fairly accurate) a high/dangerous SNAP score is less than 50 percent accurate as a predictor of death, and the score might be "more useful as an epidemiological measure of outcomes for large groups of babies than . . . as a clinical guide to treatment decisions for an individual baby."[16]

Rather skeptical of quantitative measures like this, Lantos finally considers an interesting predictive option: the clinical intuitions of NICU workers. He asked NICU workers to make a daily judgment whether 333 very sick infants (each weighing less than 1,000 grams or on mechanical ventilation) would live or die. Every physician on *every* day predicted that 231 of these babies would live; remarkably, they all did live. However, for the other 102 NICU babies, the clinicians were neither uniformly optimistic nor uniformly accurate. About half of these babies were predicted by all caregivers on each day to die — and they were again all correct. However, clinicians' intuitions were not always the same. Babies whom every clinician predicted to die, on at least

---

14. Lantos and Meadow, *Neonatal Bioethics*, 92.
15. Lantos and Meadow, *Neonatal Bioethics*, 93.
16. Lantos and Meadow, *Neonatal Bioethics*, 95.

*one* day, often did not die. In addition, of the babies who had at least one day on which two or more clinicians predicted death a full one-third survived. Also surviving were one-fourth of the babies who, on at least one day, were predicted by *all* the clinicians to die. Though perhaps more helpful than one might suppose, clinical intuition certainly has its predictive limits.

However, there are other important predictive factors to take into account that neither Lantos nor the SNAP score considers. A study commissioned by the National Institute of Child Health and Human Development Neonatal Research Network found that factoring in things like sex, exposure or nonexposure to antenatal corticosteroids, and single or multiple gestation can make outcome predictions significantly more accurate. Remarkably, "In multivariable models of infants who received intensive care, female sex, exposure to antenatal corticosteroid therapy, singleton birth, and increased birth weight (per 100-g increment) were each associated with benefits similar to those of an increase in gestational age of approximately 1 week."[17] This usually means a very significant decrease in mortality, morbidity, and use of resources.

Of particular interest is the role that sex plays in predicting outcomes. The study found that babies at twenty-three weeks gestation, weighing between 401 and 500 grams, survived at a remarkably different rate depending on whether the baby was male or female. Males had an 8 percent observed rate of survival without profound impairment. But females had a 19 percent observed rate of survival without profound impairment. A 50 percent improvement in outcomes is unique to this specific age and weight class, but multiple studies have found a broad trend of females doing 10-20 percent better than males across the board.[18]

Especially in light of the amazing story of Amelia Sonja Taylor — a black preterm girl who survived after being born at twenty-one weeks six days gestation (cited in the introduction to this book) — much has been made of the role *race* plays as a predictive factor as well. Despite

17. Jon E. Tyson et al., "Intensive Care for Extreme Prematurity — Moving beyond Gestational Age," *New England Journal of Medicine* 358 (April 2008): 1679.

18. For instance: Timothy R. La Pine, J. Craig Jackson, and F. C. Bennett, "Outcome of Infants Weighing Less Than 800 Grams at Birth: 15 Years' Experience," *Pediatrics* 96 (1995), and Steven B. Morse et al., "Racial and Gender Differences in the Viability of Extremely Low Birth Weight Infants: A Population-Based Study" (2006).

many studies with data to the contrary, the Tyson study found that "In bivariable analyses as well as analyses adjusted for the center and the factors described above, race or ethnic group had no significant association with outcomes."[19] This flies in the face of the data of several other studies, including the Morse study cited below. Though they admit that the issue of black race conferring a survival advantage has been debated, they find that

> black race conferred a significant survival advantage at 1 year of age across all gestational ages among ELBW [extremely low-birth-weight] infants. The steepest part of the survival curves in Figs 2 and 3 occurred among the lower birth weights and gestational ages, indicating increasing advantage of black race as the degree of prematurity increases. In addition, the OR for black versus white survival was 1.3 (95% CI:1.1–1.5), favoring black race. Our results suggest that race plays an important role in estimates of survival rates and therefore may affect treatment decisions.[20]

As dramatic as these numbers are — they show that being black is an even better boon to an NICU baby than being female — they are nothing compared to when one *combines* race and sex. The Morse study found that when "Combining race and gender, the largest advantage was seen among black female infants, compared with white male infants, with a 2.1 (95% CI: 1.7–2.6) increased odds of survival."[21] In light of these numbers, (1) it is hardly surprising that baby Taylor was the first to break into the twenty-one-week survivor category, and (2) race and gender should at least be candidates for factors to use when predicting NICU outcomes. This will become important in determining the final constructive proposal of book.

## The "Culture" of the NICU

All this discussion cannot, however, neglect the social context or "culture" in which NICU treatment decisions take place. One might think

19. Tyson et al., "Intensive Care," 1679.
20. Morse et al., "Racial and Gender Differences," e111.
21. Morse et al., "Racial and Gender Differences," e110.

that the place to start in exploring the culture of the NICU would be with the attitudes and practices of physicians and other clinicians. But it seems clear that — especially in light of the shift to patient and parental autonomy in the twentieth century — we should first briefly look at attitudes and practices of parents if we want a comprehensive understanding of the culture of the NICU.

The overwhelming majority of parents in the NICU want their babies to survive and will often demand that "everything be done" to save them. This is true for a number of reasons. First, it just seems that parents, happily, simply have an innate love for their children and want to see them survive so that they can continue to love them. Second, a good number of babies in the NICU are there precisely due to "multiple birth" complications — and these are often the result of IVF and implantation. Such parents are often quite desperate to have a child: both from a psychological and a financial point of view. Third, a significant number of parents bring a religious view into the NICU that God requires them to "do everything they can" for their baby; otherwise they are "killing" her. Since only God can be the author of life and death, they have a strict duty as parents to err on the side of life and put the rest into God's hands.[22] Nearly every neonatologist one speaks with confirms this generalization. An article in the *Boston Globe* exploring parental attitudes toward NICU treatments, for instance, claimed the following: "But mostly the doctor's warnings are met with blank stares, or even anger, and expectant parents choose to hold on to the hope that they will hit the prematurity jackpot and take home a relatively normal baby. 'I have come to the conclusion,' admits Fiascone [a Tufts Medical Center neonatologist], 'that even when you explain to parents that the chance of survival without major injury is a very low percentage, most of them still want you to do everything you can to resuscitate their baby.'"[23]

That these attitudes of the parents contribute to a "culture of overtreatment" in the NICU is borne out by the sociological literature. For instance, Guillemin and Holmstrom argue that "Parents' sheer de-

---

22. It is certainly worth noting here that, if one accepts the Christian tradition on ordinary and extraordinary means detailed in chapter 2, this view is fundamentally mistaken.

23. Adam Wolfberg, "Extreme Preemies," *Boston Globe,* April 27, 2008.

termination coupled with their commitment to the survival of their infant . . . contributed to the aggressiveness of treatment in the n.i.c.u."[24]

But the culture of overtreatment in the NICU is not simply the result of parental attitudes and decisions. Physicians play a major role as well. Guillemin and Holmstrom argue that, perhaps due to the social structures of the clinical setting where "doctors are supposed to act like doctors," the most fundamental decision that contributes to the culture of the NICU — whether or not to go all out — "was easily and routinely made, and the answer was in the affirmative." They note that "the decision to be aggressive did not involve long discussion, reflection, or emotional agonizing. On the contrary, such decisions were virtually automatic."[25]

In addition to the rigid and isolated roles and structure of the NICU, another reason physician attitudes and practices contribute to a culture of overtreatment is that a significant number of neonatologists will err on the side of performing the tasks for which they have been trained — especially when success would mean prestige for them among their colleagues. William Silverman, one of the "grandfathers" of neonatology, described precisely this attitude in himself.[26] As a young physician in the 1940s, Silverman was given the opportunity to treat an ELBW infant about whom he admitted the following: almost no babies of this age ever survived. If the baby did somehow survive he had no idea about the long-term outlook for the child. If she had been born in another building she would been considered "pre-viable" and simply would have been allowed to die. Nevertheless, Silverman — without getting consent from the baby's parents — gave the child aggressive treatment. He not only used the standard procedures, but went so far as to *transfuse his own blood* into his patient in order to overcome a defect of blood gas transport. Of this move, Silverman says:

> This optimistic suggestion for an untried treatment was just the kind of bold action I was looking for. I began to transfuse the infant daily with a few millimeters of my own blood. I quickly became con-

24. Jeanne Harley Guillemin and Lynda Lytle Holmstrom, *Mixed Blessings: Intensive Care for Newborns* (New York: Oxford University Press, 1986), 139.

25. Guillemin and Holmstrom, *Mixed Blessings*, 114-15.

26. W. A. Silverman, "Overtreatment of Neonates? A Personal Retrospective," *Pediatrics* 90 (1992): 971.

vinced that it was my carbonic-anhydrase-rich blood that was keeping this baby alive — and I was not unmindful of the fact that she
was setting a new hospital record for longevity! Now, was this
*overtreatment*. . . ? The question never entered my head! And it never
seemed to occur to my teachers. The baby was presented at grand
rounds as a triumph of mechanism-guided treatment, and I was
made to feel like a hero. My rescue fantasy was fulfilled.[27]

Modern-day grand rounds in research hospitals with an NICU suggest
that little has changed with regard to these kinds of stories today.

But a third factor most certainly contributes to the attitudes and
practices of physicians in the NICU: the law. Or, perhaps better, clinical
perception or fear of the law. Prior to the 1980s, claims Norm Fost,
courts were generally supportive of decisions to remove life-sustaining
and curative treatment of neonates who had Down syndrome and
spina bifida. This was true even "when it was implausible that withholding treatment was in the child's interests."[28] This all changed with
the case of Baby Doe — an infant with Down syndrome and esophageal
atresia who was refused a common and likely successful treatment because the parents decided that a Down syndrome life was not worth living. The Reagan administration, spurred on by disability rights and
pro-life groups, cracked down on states receiving federal funding by,
with limited exceptions,[29] demanding that NICUs provide medically
necessary treatment regardless of mental disability. Otherwise clinicians and hospitals would be subject to prosecution under federal child
abuse statutes and loss of federal support. Some NICUs even had red
phones in them that had direct lines to federal authorities to be used to
report any Baby Doe–type situations being considered and executed.

The result of this shift, says Fost, is that a "prolonged history of
what is now perceived as serious undertreatment of infants with reasonable prospects for living a meaningful life was replaced by an era of serious overtreatment. One form of child abuse, neglect, was replaced by a

27. Silverman, "Overtreatment of Neonates?" 971.

28. Norm Fost, "Decisions regarding Treatment of Seriously Ill Newborns," *Journal of the American Medical Association* 281 (1999): 2041.

29. Exceptions were allowed for infants in an irreversible coma, for treatments that were futile, and for treatments that were "inhumane," although the definition of that term has been the subject of continuing controversy.

form of medical battering."[30] John Lantos suggests that the legal situation is such that doctors today simply don't want to risk "what a judge might say" and thus might say to a child's parents, for instance, "It is considered child abuse not to operate on your baby's intestinal blockage, even though the baby has Down syndrome." Most parents do not want to be charged with child abuse and to face a legal proceeding they know they will lose, so they agree to the surgery and do not go to court. In such cases, the law has an effect even though the effect is not measurable through the frequency of its use.[31] Indeed, the law seems to have had an effect even beyond what it actually was intended to do. In a study called *The Appleton Consensus*[32] — convened by an international group of physicians, ethicists, and medical economists — it was found that

> U.S. neonatologists widely agree that the [Baby Doe] law is believed to require overtreatment of infants, and this results in practice in many terminally ill infants receiving inappropriately aggressive care for long periods. This is an inaccurate interpretation of what the law requires. Current U.S. Federal law simply mandates that states that wish to receive Federal grants for child abuse and neglect services must have in place a mechanism to review suspected cases of "medical neglect." No treatment of infants is mandated by that law and no penalties against physicians, parents, or hospitals for non-treatment are contained within the law. . . . If U.S. neonatologists employ overly aggressive treatment, they cannot blame it on the current state of U.S. law.[33]

Lantos also notes something essential about Baby Doe and the NICU "culture" (legal and otherwise): "After the Baby Doe controversy, in which the federal government tried to mandate the treatment of almost all newborns, it became difficult to imagine a public policy in the United States that would allow care to be systematically limited. Instead, the opposite happened. Public policies were enacted that generously reimbursed NICUs."[34] This fact will become especially important when considering the economics of the NICU.

30. Fost, "Decisions regarding Treatment," 2041.

31. Lantos and Meadow, *Neonatal Bioethics*, 82-83.

32. J. M. Stanley, *The Appleton Consensus: Suggested International Guidelines for Decisions to Forego Medical Treatment*, vol. 15 (London: British Medical Association, 1989), 129.

33. Stanley, *The Appleton Consensus*, 18.

34. Lantos and Meadow, *Neonatal Bioethics*, 129.

This culture of overtreatment does not exist uniformly around the world, but is especially strong in the United States. In another international study, this one about neonatologists' attitudes and practices in Europe, it was found that while making a decision to withhold or withdraw life-sustaining treatment based on "poor neurological prognosis" grounds "raises issues of discrimination against the disabled, as the American 'Baby Doe' regulations clearly point out," this was not a significant moral distinction in the majority of European countries studied. Indeed, "the proportion of physicians involved, at least once in the course of their professional life, in decisions to forego treatment because of poor neurological prognosis is very close to that for fatal and terminal conditions."[35]

We now attempt to show how this culture of overtreatment in the American NICU has a direct economic impact on both the NICU and the wider health care system in the United States — and that such an impact is open to serious critique from Catholic social teaching.

## Economic Considerations

Finding out how much we spend in the NICU in the United States is not an easy business. Private insurance companies (who have no public reporting requirements) pay for a large share of the care, but so does Medicaid — and because Medicaid is administered by states with their own rules and regulations, it is difficult to estimate total costs even with public reporting. Lantos attempts to estimate it by taking a study of twenty-five NICUs from 1993-94 and adjusting for modern-day numbers.[36] He suggests that "the direct cost of NICUs in the United States in 2004 could be estimated at about $21 billion."[37]

35. Marina Cuttini, *Ethical Issues in Neonatal Intensive Care and Physicians' Practices: A European Perspective* (Oslo: Scandinavian University Press, 2006), 44.

36. In his adjustment he simply assumes that the numbers of NICU admissions are about the same ten years later — but gives us no reason to accept this assumption. Given the increase in IVF, multiple births, and the corresponding ELBW babies — to say nothing of the dramatic increase in NICUs (which he himself cites a few pages later) — this is very little reason to accept it. And there is very good reason to think that the total cost is higher, and perhaps substantially so.

37. Lantos and Meadow, *Neonatal Bioethics*, 124.

But what about more specific cost information relevant to this book? A 2005 study that looked at data from several hundred thousand live births in California found that "costs increase dramatically with decreasing birth-weight. Average total hospital costs for infants who weighed 2000-2499 g at birth were ~$1200 compared with average hospital costs of nearly $119,000 for infants who weighed 1000 to 1249 g at birth."[38] This was due in part to "increasing use of advanced medical technologies and complex medical and surgical procedures," but it also was affected by longer hospital stays in general. For babies with a birth weight between 750 and 999 grams, their median length of stay was 71.0 days. For babies with a birth weight over 2,500 grams, the median length of stay was 2.0 days. The median daily cost for those in the former category was $2,380 with a median total cost per stay of $165,248. By contrast, the median daily cost for those in the latter category was $316 with a median total cost per stay of $570.[39] Costs for low-birth-weight babies "make up a hugely disproportionate share" of the total hospital costs for infants. Consider that very low-birth-weight infants accounted for only 0.9 percent of the cases, but for a whopping 35.7 percent of the costs. Low-birth-weight infants account for only 5.9 percent of the cases but a dramatic 56.6 percent of the costs. It is simply remarkable that only about 7 percent of the cases account for over 90 percent of the total costs.

The California study is self-consciously aware that it is dealing only with premature deliveries, but also notes that "congenital anomalies are another significant cause of neonatal costs, and most of these infants are term deliveries. . . . [And] in a simple classification of the cases with major congenital anomalies, they represent a similar disproportionate share of neonatal hospital costs."[40] A report from the Centers for Disease Control and Prevention outlines some of the NICU data with respect to specific birth defects in some detail.[41] The average length of stay was longest for those babies with surgically repaired

38. Susan K. Schmitt, "Costs of Newborn Care in California: A Population-Based Study," *Pediatrics* 117 (2006): 159.

39. Schmitt, "Costs of Newborn Care," 157.

40. Schmitt, "Costs of Newborn Care," 159.

41. Centers for Disease Control and Prevention, "Hospital Stays, Hospital Charges, and In-Hospital Deaths among Infants with Selected Birth Defects — United States, 2003" (2007).

gastroschisis: 41.0 days. Other numbers of note included spina bifida: 15.1; pulmonary valve stenosis: 22.8; esophageal atresia: 31.3; Down syndrome: 11.1; trisomy 13/18: 7.7/10.2. The most expensive NICU charges were for two congenital heart defects: hypoplastic left heart at $199,597 and common truncus ateriousus at $192,781. Other cost numbers of interest included: spina bifida: $65,342; pulmonary valve stenosis: $80,814; esophageal atresia: $136,631; Down syndrome: $38,745; and trisomy 13/18: $30,021/$39,547.[42]

These numbers have the power to produce strong reactions all by themselves. But, of course, they do not exist in a contextless socioeconomic vacuum — and locating them in that context makes them even more powerful. Though not necessarily the same as today's NICU reality,[43] M. H. Shearer provided the context for such numbers at the beginning of the 1980s. She pointed out that even though the nursery and labor/delivery unit had traditionally been loss leaders in hospital accounting, the reimbursement rates of Medicaid, Handicapped Children's Services, and Blue-Cross/Blue-Shield in the NICU were much higher and actually made the NICU a profit center for a hospital. One result of this was an 18 percent increase in the number of NICUs with concomitant reduction in newborn nursery space. Another result was that in order to match the professionally required occupancy rate for NICU beds, mildly sick or, in rare cases, even healthy newborns were admitted.[44] Lantos also cites numbers from the 1980s that confirm this. The NICU at Stanford University, for instance, though it comprised only 3.7 percent of the total hospital beds, generated 4.7 percent of the revenue for the hospital. In addition, 82 percent of the faculty-generated revenue for patient care in the department of pediatrics came from the NICU — subsidizing the entire department and, to some extent, the entire hospital.[45]

Lantos argues that these trends continue today in part because the NICU is one of the few areas in which inpatient activity is increasing rather than decreasing. (Recall the numbers with regard to average hospital stays cited above.) Indeed, he goes even further and makes the following dramatic claim: "The NICU has become the economic engine

42. Centers for Disease Control and Prevention, "Hospital Stays," 28.
43. Though it will become clear later that it is much the same.
44. M. H. Shearer, "The Economics of Intensive-Care for the Full-Term Newborn," *Birth* 7, no. 4 (1980): 234.
45. Lantos and Meadow, *Neonatal Bioethics*, 130.

that keeps our children's hospitals running. The survival of hospital-based pediatrics as we know it is increasingly dependent on continued commitment to the technologies and the personnel that enable the survival of extremely premature babies." In support of this claim he cites his own University of Chicago Hospital (UCH), which he claims, though it accounted for only 4 percent of the patients in the hospital in 2002, accounted for 10 percent of the revenue. Put another way, "the total operating margin of UCH in that year was $23.8 million. Of that, $11.4 million, or 48%, came from the NICU."[46]

Another trend that continues today is NICU building in relationship to hospital strategic planning. In an effort to boost profitability, NICU building continues at a rapid pace. Lantos notes that his own UCH, due in part to NICU profitability, was able to build a brand-new children's hospital in 2005 — with, of course, 10 percent more NICU beds. He also cites a hospital in Boston that on August 30, 2002, had its bond rating downgraded "due to the hospital's declining operating performance." On November 20, 2002, it was reported that the hospital was building a ten-bed NICU — making it the first nonteaching hospital in the state to do so.[47]

A third trend that continues is the number of NICU beds outpacing need and questionable practices in order to deal with this problem. Lantos cites a study that showed that from 1980 to 1995 the number of hospitals grew by 99 percent, the number of NICU beds by 138 percent, and the number of neonatologists by 268 percent. By contrast, the growth in needed NICU bed days was only 84 percent. A study appearing in a 2007 issue of *Pediatrics* found that when the NICU census "was in the highest quintile, patients were 32% more likely to be discharged when compared with all of the other quintiles of unit census." However, when the NICU census "was in the lowest quintile, patients were 20% less likely to be discharged when compared with all of the other quintiles of unit census."[48]

International comparisons also suggest that "proliferation of NICUs in the United States, driven by their profitability, is leading to

46. Lantos and Meadow, *Neonatal Bioethics,* 131.

47. Lantos and Meadow, *Neonatal Bioethics,* 31.

48. Jochen Profit, "Neonatal Intensive Care Unit Census Influences Discharge of Moderately Preterm Infants," *Pediatrics* (2007): 314.

profligate overuse of NICU technology."[49] For instance, the United States has 6.1 neonatologists per 1,000 live births, while Australia, Canada, and the U.K. have 3.7, 3.3, and 2.7, respectively. Better results, however, have not been produced in the United States. The relative risk, with the United States as a reference, of neonatal mortality for infants less than 1,000 grams was 0.84 for Australia, 1.12 for Canada, and 0.99 for the U.K. For infants 1,000 to 2,499 grams, the relative risk was 0.97 for Australia, 1.26 for Canada, and 0.95 for the U.K.[50]

## NICU Attitudes and Practices: A Critique

The first part of this chapter marshaled evidence that there is a "culture of overtreatment" in American neonatal intensive care units. Let us review the major factors contributing to this culture:

1. The attitude and perspective of parents who most often "want everything done." (This is sometimes based on a misunderstanding of the Christian tradition on withdrawal and refusal of treatment.)
2. The institutionalization of NICU treatments. "Doctors act like doctors." "Nurses act like nurses." And so on. Health care professionals simply treat illness. They are neither trained nor encouraged to take broader goods into consideration.
3. The prestige and ego factor. Some neonatologists admit that this is a motivation in some cases of overtreatment.
4. The law: both in its indirect perception and in its direct application. Many clinicians (wrongly) believe that the Baby Doe regulation and what has followed demand that they engage in treatment behaviors that contribute to a NICU culture of overtreatment.
5. NICU treatment profitability. The market helps to contribute to the culture of treatment as well.

This culture of overtreatment has led to

NICU treatment that is disproportionate with much of the rest of health care expenditures in the United States. This is especially true

49. Lantos and Meadow, *Neonatal Bioethics,* 134.
50. Lantos and Meadow, *Neonatal Bioethics,* 134.

when one considers the share of resources allotted to low-birth-weight babies and babies with congenital anomalies. Also of note is the dramatic increase in new NICUs and the number of neonatology specialists.

Chapters 2 and 3 already gave us one direct critique of this situation. Even when we are considering the "individualistically narrow" best interests of the imperiled newborn, the culture of overtreatment in the NICU sometimes (and perhaps often) loses those considerations in favor of some of the considerations mentioned above. And the Christian tradition on ordinary/extraordinary means supports such a critique. But what chapter 3 attempted to show was that this critique can and should go wider and deeper — with a much broader understanding of what it means to talk about what is in someone's "best interests." It is to this broader critique we now turn.

## Catholic Social Teaching and the "Culture of Overtreatment" in the NICU

The first thing Catholic social teaching demands is that we look at the NICU culture of treatment in the broader health care context in which it takes place.[51] The United States, despite spending nearly $2 trillion on health care annually (far and away the highest in the world — even as a percentage of GDP), still allows many millions (even factoring in health care reform) to go without health insurance. In addition, anywhere from 15 to 49 million more are underinsured: those with medical needs not covered by their insurance, medical needs that are covered but with high co-payments that force beneficiaries to forgo or delay treatment, or out-of-pocket health care expenditures in excess of 10 percent of their income. Programs designed to help the poor in this regard — primarily state-run Medicaid programs — are not solvent and (as we saw with TennCare in chapter 3) are often forced to drop even those with life-threatening conditions. Those without health insur-

---

51. Of course, it will also demand that we look at other social contexts: worldwide health care problems, other resource-allocation contexts, etc. Even though these are important questions, they go beyond the scope of this book. It is certainly an area for future work and study.

ance, or who are forced to delay treatment, are four times more likely to require avoidable hospitalization and emergency room treatment for conditions like diabetes, asthma, hypertension, and pneumonia — as well as being far more likely to be diagnosed with late-stage cancer. All this culminates in the United States lagging far behind other countries — many of which spend dramatically less on health care — on important health metrics like life expectancy, infant mortality, obesity, and other morbidity rates.[52]

We have already seen that the anthropology of Catholic social teaching (CST) is such that a human person is fundamentally and intrinsically social. This can be described in theologically "thick" ways (such as by appealing to human beings having been made in the image of an essentially relational, triune God) or with simple appeals to the empirical fact of our multiplied social interconnections — especially in light of a globalized world. John Paul II reminds us that our fundamental sociality implies a duty of solidarity in which "all really are responsible for all." On what should this duty focus? Recall the "first principle" of CST:

> The right to the common use of goods is "the first principle of the whole ethical and social order" and "the characteristic principle of Christian social doctrine" . . . it is innate in individual persons, in every person, and has *priority* with regard to any human intervention concerning goods, to any legal system concerning the same, to any economic or social system or method: "All other rights, whatever they are, including property rights and the right of free trade must be subordinated to this norm [the universal destination of goods]; they must not hinder it, but rather expedite its application."[53]

What one means by a duty to promote the common use of goods needs further explanation. Drew Christiansen has argued that "the common good, as John XXIII understands it, demands keeping broad inequalities in check."[54] But also recall that one's response to inequality

52. Catholic Health Association of the United States, "Continuing the Commitment: A Pathway to Health Care Reform" (April 2000).

53. Pontificium Consilium de Iustitia et Pace, *Compendium of the Social Doctrine of the Church* (Dublin: Veritas, 2005), 82; hereafter Pontifical Council, *Compendium*.

54. Kenneth R. Himes and Lisa Cahill, *Modern Catholic Social Teaching: Commentaries and Interpretations* (Washington, D.C.: Georgetown University Press, 2005), 228.

cannot simply be to distribute goods equally without social context. No, the concept of equality — at least since the social teaching of Pope Paul VI — is directly connected to *participation*. He says: "While scientific and technological progress continues to overturn man's surroundings, his patterns of knowledge, work, consumption, and relationships, two aspirations persistently make themselves felt in these new contexts, and they grow stronger to the extent that he becomes better informed and better educated: the aspiration to equality and the aspiration to participation, two forms of man's dignity and freedom."[55]

The U.S. bishops would build on Paul VI's understanding of the relationship between equality and participation by claiming that justice demands "the establishment of minimum levels of participation in the life of the human community for all persons," and that "social institutions be ordered in a way that guarantees all persons the ability to participate actively in the economic, political, and cultural life of society."[56]

In determining whether attitudes and practices in the American NICU are proportionate with the common good, then, we have to ask about its relationship to the ability of all persons to "actively participate" — and in this context, to actively participate (at a minimum level, at least) in the life of the health care community. The "culture of overtreatment" in the NICU — when looked at as a whole — certainly has produced lots of participation: 1.6 million life-years added each year. However, when we look at more specific aspects of NICU treatments, its relationship to participation becomes much cloudier — especially if we look at NICU babies with extremely low birth weights and with certain kinds of congenital anomalies. Such babies make up a very small proportion of a hospital patient census but require a shockingly disproportionate share of medical resources. This is true simply on the level of individual payments considered at a particular point in time. But it is even more worryingly disproportionate when one considers the economic results that such treatments produce, namely, a dramatic and disproportionate shift of limited health care resources to imperiled newborns and

55. Paul VI, *Octogesima Adveniens* (New York: Paulist, 1971), 22.

56. National Conference of Catholic Bishops, *Economic Justice for All: Pastoral Letter on Catholic Social Teaching and the U.S. Economy*, vol. 101 (Washington, D.C.: Office of Publishing and Promotion Services, United States Catholic Conference, 1986), 78.

away from others who are often without even a "basic minimum" level of participation in the American health care system.

A major reason why such a culture of overtreatment in the NICU exists at such variance with the common good is because of the kinds of social structures that underlie such treatment: the individual-istically narrow roles of neonatal clinicians, technological idolization, hiring and promotion of medical researchers and professors, stacked legal rulings and the culture of health care litigiousness, and the mar-ket forces involved in health care. The United States bishops, when talking specifically about health care, have this issue at the center of their discussion. Our duty of solidarity requires us to "correct any un-just social, political and economic structures and institutions which are the causes of suffering."[57] John Paul II goes so far as to call such structures *sinful*:

> If the present situation can be attributed to difficulties of various kinds, it is not out of place to speak of "structures of sin" which . . . are rooted in personal sin and thus always linked to the concrete acts of individuals who introduce these structures, consolidate them, and make them difficult to remove. And thus they grow stronger, spread, and become the source of other sins, and so influence peo-ple's behavior. "Sin" and "structures of sin" are categories which are seldom applied to the situation of the contemporary world. How-ever, one cannot easily gain a profound understanding of the reality that confronts us unless we give a name to the root of the evils which afflict us.[58]

Catholic social teaching is particularly aware of two kinds of sinful social structures, both of which are related to each other: the "techno-logical imperative" and the unrestrained free market. It is supremely aware that

> The present historical period has placed at the disposal of society new goods that were completely unknown until recent times. This

57. National Conference of Catholic Bishops, "U.S. Bishops' Pastoral Letter on Healthcare" (1981), 297.

58. John Paul II, *Sollicitudo Rei Socialis* (Washington, D.C.: Office of Publishing and Promotion Services, United States Catholic Conference, 1988), 36.

calls for a fresh reading of the principle of the universal destination of goods of the earth and makes it necessary to extend this principle so that it includes the latest developments brought about by economic and technological progress. . . . New technological and scientific knowledge must be placed at the service of mankind's primary needs, gradually increasing humanity's common patrimony.[59]

Catholic social teaching warns that any social structure where use of technology is an "end in itself" (554) is sinful because it does not take into account the ultimate end of these and all goods. Technologies, "like all goods, have a *universal destination;* they too must be placed in a context of legal norms and social rules that guarantee that they will be used according to the criteria of justice, equity and respect of human rights" (283). Insofar as NICU treatments drive a technological imperative that is unaware of — or even antithetical to — a universal destination of goods aimed at equality of participation in the health care community, they are part of a sinful social structure that works against the common good.

The other sinful social structure — which no doubt drives some of the technological imperative — is a free market without due regulation. While private property is a "highly necessary" sphere and "ought to be considered part of an extension of human freedom," it is "in its essence only an instrument for respecting the principle of the universal destination of goods; in the final analysis therefore, it is not an end but a means" (176-77). The market's regulation of such property is an "irreplaceable instrument" for an economic system, but most certainly needs to be disciplined by "ethical objectives." To do this, one must be aware that the market alone cannot be entrusted with the task of supplying every category of goods — for some goods, by their very nature, are not and cannot be mere commodities. This is easily seen "in [the market's] proven inability to satisfy important human needs" (349). One of these needs, most certainly, is health care. And in this context one can see quite clearly how the sinful social structure of the improperly regulated market works in the culture of treatment in the NICU: the profitability of such treatments drives resources toward imperiled

59. Pontifical Council, *Compendium,* 179. In-text references in the following few paragraphs are to page numbers in this document.

newborns — and away from other needy patients — in a way that is disproportionate with the common good.


## Catholic Social Teaching on Solutions to the Problem

If NICU treatments of certain imperiled newborns are indeed disproportionate with the common good,[60] what suggestions does Catholic social teaching have for dealing with this problem? It is self-consciously aware of its limitations for *technical* solutions and therefore does not "propose or establish systems or models of social organization" (68). However, it does give some broad outlines and principles to use in dealing with these kinds of problems. At a most basic level, the market and state are to act in concert and complement each other, with the state organized in such a manner that it gives an ethical direction to economic development. Because equality, and therefore participation, should be at the heart of such direction, it becomes necessary for the state to regulate "certain sectors of the market" that are "not able to guarantee an equitable distribution of goods and services that are essential for the human growth of its citizens" (353). The public authorities, in this context, are "called to carry out substantial reforms of economic, political, cultural and technological structures and the necessary changes in institutions" (197). For, "If it is true that everyone is born with the right to use the goods of the earth, it is likewise true that, in order to ensure that this right is exercised in an equitable and orderly fashion, regulated interventions are necessary, interventions that are the result of national . . . agreements." Equality and solidarity are explicitly invoked in this context as essential principles for informing "redistribution of resources" and "public spending" (173 and 355).

About the disproportionate treatments resulting from a culture of overtreatment in the NICU, then, Catholic social teaching argues for regulation by the public authorities aimed at the common good, equality, and participation. This becomes even more morally urgent given the health care crisis described above. As Joseph Boyle argues, in cases of "systematic scarcity [which describes our health care system more

60. And the book is a long way from having shown this — more counterarguments will be dealt with later in this chapter.

generally] someone in authority in a community or institutional system must decide that some resources will be directed to meeting certain needs of community members, and as a result become unavailable to meet other needs of all or some in the community." Indeed, "One purpose of authority in Catholic Social Teaching is to coordinate the actions of individuals so they can cooperate for common goods. The need for the kind of social choice authority makes possible is especially urgent when moral problems emerge that cannot possibly be solved by the uncoordinated actions of even the most conscientious individuals and small communities."[61]

These hard choices need to take place in a realistic context — a context that understands that human needs, whether medical or otherwise, will always outstrip resources. This is the nature of the finite beings we are and the finite world in which we live. As Mark Cherry argues, all health care — and not just NICU treatment — "is provided within the conditions of human finitude. It is false to assume that all can be provided equal care, the very best of care, with physician and patient choice, without rationing, while still managing to control costs . . . such a view, however prevalent, fails to face the economic, medical and moral realities of healthcare. It represents an ideology, a false consciousness, which all economic indicators and empirical experiences show to be false, but the reality of which few are willing to openly confront."[62] This book attempts to use the resources of Catholic social teaching to openly confront the sinful social structures present in the culture of overtreatment in the NICU — and the uncomfortable conclusions that may follow from addressing them.

## An "Asked and Answered" Rejoinder?

If one had not read chapters 2 and 3 of this book, one might take this conclusion to be absurd on its face. Surely the duty of medical personnel in the NICU — or anywhere else — cannot include such broad con-

---

61. H. Tristram Engelhardt and Mark J. Cherry, *Allocating Scarce Medical Resources: Roman Catholic Perspectives*, Clinical Medical Ethics Series (Washington, D.C.: Georgetown University Press, 2002), 88.

62. Engelhardt and Cherry, *Allocating Scarce Medical Resources*, 20.

siderations of economic justice; surely their duty is to the patient in front of them. Limiting neonatal treatment will force clinicians to abandon patients in a way that flies in the face of the very foundation of medicine and is a clear affront to human dignity.

But recall the response to these worries in chapters 2 and 3. Clinicians, if they are really acting in the best interests of their patients, cannot treat patients in social isolation — as if one's good could be socially separated from the good of others. No, part of what it means to act in the best interests of a patient is to offer treatments consistent with the common good and refuse treatments that are disproportionate with it. Hardly an affront to human dignity or the foundations of medicine, this is exactly the kind of reasoning used in triage medicine — when medical need most clearly and directly outstrips resources. There the choice is not between "abandoning" and "not abandoning" — but rather *how* and *on what basis* persons (with full moral status) will be "abandoned." Given the problems of our health care system mentioned above, it is simply a "hard truth" that we are in a tragic triage situation already. We are abandoning patients *right now*. The question is, Are we going to continue to abandon them in a way that our sinful social structures demand — or are we going to do what the common good demands? These are difficult questions, but this is no reason for not openly confronting them. The stakes are about as high as they can get.

Perhaps one reason why some fail to see the applicability of triage reasoning with regard to our health care system is because the analogy fails. In a real triage situation, the resources (whether time, hospital beds, ventilators, vaccines, etc.) in play are all being used for the needy patient community in question: a battlefield, a disaster area, etc. When resources are limited for some patients in the community, it is because they will go directly to the other needy patients. Perhaps this is analogous to single-payer health care systems in Europe with fixed budgets, but it is less clear that this applies to the "fee for service" private system in the United States. If a battlefield medic passes over one patient, it is because her resources will be better used to serve the common good of her community elsewhere. But if the U.S. federal government were to limit neonatal treatment, say, with a system like the one in the Netherlands where no babies under twenty-five weeks will be treated, it isn't at all certain that the resources would then go to places that better serve the common good. Indeed, if the patient was covered by private insurance, the resources could go to any number of medical uses that the insurance company covers: hip replacements, Viagra, acid reflux, and hundreds of other maladies that would not proportionally serve the common good.[63] If the U.S. health care system isn't analogous to a triage situation, why use triage reasoning to support proposed reforms?

Not all the proposed reforms in the final part of this chapter are dependent on the triage analogy. Even if the analogy does not work, the sinful social structures still exist in the system and some practical remedies will be suggested that have nothing whatever to do with triage reasoning. But we do have something like a single-payer system, often with a fixed budget, for health care delivery: Medicaid. Let us take a more detailed look at the program to see if the triage analogy — and resulting critique — does in fact follow.[64]

## Medicaid

The largest growth in an entitlement program in the United States during the last part of the twentieth century was to be found in Medicaid.[65] In 1984 the Medicaid program spent $38 billion, 4.4 percent of the federal budget, accounted for 0.97 percent of GDP, and covered 22 million persons. In 1999 the program spent $172 billion, 9.7 percent of the federal budget, accounted for 1.9 percent of GDP, and covered 38 million persons. This growth is even more remarkable given a nearly parallel rise in the numbers of nonelderly persons without health insurance — the major part of the population Medicaid was designed to serve.

63. It is also a distinct possibility that much of the saved resources would go into the pockets of the insurance company's shareholders.

64. What follows is a description of the Medicaid program as this book goes to press. The United States is considering expanding and changing the Medicaid system in a way that will make rationing even more explicit and necessary — and thus the central argument of this book even more relevant.

65. The background information on Medicaid will, for the most part, come from Jonathan Gruber and the National Bureau of Economic Research, *Medicaid*, NBER Working Paper Series, no. 7829 (Cambridge, Mass.: National Bureau of Economic Research, 2000), 101; http://www.nber.org/papers/W7829.pdf; hereafter Gruber and NBER, *Medicaid*.

Medicaid is actually four public insurance programs in one that serves four groups of needy patients. It provides:

1. Coverage of most medical expenses for low-income women and children.
2. Coverage of supplemental portions of medical expenditures not covered by Medicare for the low-income elderly.
3. Coverage of most medical expenses for the low-income disabled.
4. Payment of nursing home expenditures for many of the institutionalized elderly.

The first function encompasses about two-thirds of the program's enrollees, while the last three functions encompass about one-third.[66]

Though the federal government puts significant resources into Medicaid, each state administers its own program with some discretion to be balanced against federal regulation and oversight by the Health Care Financing Administration and the Department of Health and Human Services. But in general the program is designed to provide health care to the very poor in the groups mentioned above, though the states have significant leeway when determining eligibility criteria — which are usually based on some baseline related to a federal- or state-determined poverty level.

Though states have some significant freedom to determine eligibility, they have much less discretion when it comes to covered services. Generally, all enrollees are mandatorily entitled to the following:[67]

- inpatient hospital services
- outpatient hospital services
- rural health clinic services
- federally qualified health center services
- laboratory and X-ray services
- nursing facility services for individuals twenty-one or older
- early and periodic screening, diagnosis, and treatment (EPSDT) services for individuals under age twenty-one
- family planning services

66. Gruber and NBER, *Medicaid*, 1.
67. Gruber and NBER, *Medicaid*, 11.

- physician services
- home health services for any individual entitled to nursing facility care
- nurse-midwife services
- services of certified nurse practitioners and certified family nurse practitioners

According to the Balanced Budget Act of 1997, however, states have full discretion to determine their own *reimbursement* plans for such services so long as they provide public notice of their proposed rates and the methods for determining those rates. Most states use:

> a purely prospective system of rates that either pay a fixed amount per day, or for the entire stay for a given diagnosis, while some states use a hybrid of retrospective and prospective reimbursement. Some states also negotiate rates with hospitals through a bidding process, whereby the states restrict enrollees' choice of hospital, and negotiate with hospitals for the right to provide services to Medicaid enrollees. In 1990, the American Hospital Association estimated that, on average, Medicaid reimburses hospitals for roughly 80% of their costs.[68]

All providers are required to accept Medicaid payment rates as payment in full. When one combines the dramatic rise in Medicaid enrollment and spending[69] with the fact that Medicaid reimburses at a significantly lesser rate than does private insurance, "providers are often reluctant to treat Medicaid patients, thus reducing the value of their coverage." Indeed, the Physician Payment Review Commission found that thirty-eight states identified low fee reimbursement as the major cause of low physician participation rates. For instance, a large body of research suggests that "increasing the ratio of Medicaid fees relative to private sector fees will increase physician participation in the program."[70]

This kind of increase would appear to have a direct impact on in-

---

68. Gruber and NBER, *Medicaid*, 13.

69. Which, importantly, is dominated by home health expenses and, in particular, home nursing. Gruber and NBER, *Medicaid*, 22.

70. Gruber and NBER, *Medicaid*, 28.

fant mortality. Projecting on the basis of data gathered from 1979 to 1992, it appears that "doubling the fee ratio would lower infant mortality by 5.2-7%."[71] In addition to reimbursement rates, Medicaid eligibility expansions also had a significant effect. For instance, during that 1979-92 period eligibility rose by 30 percent, which rise was associated with an 8.5 percent decline in the infant mortality rate. Furthermore, one could consider "targeted expansions" of Medicaid reimbursement that would deal with treatment and care directly related to imperiled newborns. Interestingly, it appears that targeted expansions work much better — at least with regard to infant mortality — than expansions that are more broad: an 11.5 percent decline in infant mortality associated with the former and only 2.9 percent with the latter. There is also "a very sizeable reduction in the incidence of low birthweight associated with targeted expansions (7.8% lower for a 30 percentage point eligibility increase), but there is no effect on low birthweight from the broad expansions."[72]

In terms of priorities when talking about reform going forward, Gruber suggests that though Medicaid eligibility expansion gets most of the attention (the State Children's Health Insurance Program [SCHIP] debates over expanding Medicaid coverage to more children being the most obvious example of this), two other areas of reform are necessary. First is "long-term care" — the largest share of Medicaid program spending. But second is Medicaid reimbursement policy. Work on physician reimbursement suggests that more generous fee schedules can lead to more access to physicians and Medicaid patients, and ultimately to better health outcomes.[73]

---

71. Gruber and NBER, *Medicaid,* 55.

72. Gruber and NBER, *Medicaid,* 51-52.

73. Gruber and NBER, *Medicaid,* 71-72. Gruber expresses frustration that more work has not been done in this area — especially given the literature that exists on Medicare reimbursement. "Variations across states, and within states over time, in Medicaid reimbursement policies offers the potential for rich investigations of how hospitals respond to reimbursement differences. Moreover, there is no work on the health impact of these hospital responses. While the state reimbursement rules may be difficult to obtain, this is clearly an interesting area for further work" (72).

## Medicaid and Triage

We can now see how the triage analogy would work with Medicaid. Each state has a single pool of money with which to work — or, perhaps in certain situations, has to view it *as if* it were a single pool in terms of controlling costs and having a workable budget. Making tough fiscal choices is essential now more than ever because — due to the dramatic increase in Medicaid costs, significantly less funding from the federal government, and mismanagement by the states — "The integrity of the Medicaid program is threatened as Medicaid budget shortfalls have occurred in more than half the states, and [were] anticipated to occur in 40 states in 2006."[74] Due to these shortfalls Medicaid budgets have to be severely limited, and therefore each state has to make triage-like decisions about who will be eligible for the program and at what rate they will reimburse for treatment to control how much is spent.

Having a relatively high reimbursement rate for NICU care — especially for the very expensive treatment of Medicaid ELBW babies and those with congenital anomalies — means that a significant number of resources are being used that cannot be used elsewhere for other Medicaid payments. And, just as in a more traditional triage situation, if NICU treatments were somehow limited, those resources *would* be available for other Medicaid payments — either as higher reimbursement rates for existing enrollees or in the form of an increased threshold for eligibility in the program. Either way, as Gruber shows, health outcomes would improve.

We could look at the patient population that is the subject of our triage reasoning in two different ways. First, we could look at treatment in proportion to the entire Medicaid population. In doing our proportional analysis of a particular NICU treatment, we would compare the good of the treatment itself with the good it could do for all Medicaid enrollees — at least in the particular state in question. Let's say Medicaid reimburses a hospital $467,567 for a baby treated in the NICU. That means there will be 467,567 fewer dollars for use, not only

74. Mary Schmeida, Ramona McNeal and Kathleen Hale, "Facing Medicaid Budget Shortfall in 2006: State Context Influences Government Health Service Cut-Backs" (paper presented at the annual meeting of the American Political Science Association, Philadelphia, August 31, 2006).

for poor babies and their mothers, but also for the low-income disabled and elderly and those in nursing homes — often for far less expensive treatments. Most obviously, this affects a state's eligibility threshold in deciding who can be a part of the program. Recall chapter 3's discussion of Tennessee's Medicaid program, which had to drop 120,000 people (many with life-threatening illnesses) due to budget shortfalls.

This, all by itself, would be enough to rethink how we apportion money in Medicaid, but consider also the quality of care for those who *are* eligible. Gruber showed us that a major reason for substandard care was the relatively low rates of physician and hospital reimbursement — which is another reality faced by states finding it necessary to control costs. An article from the *Journal of the American Medical Association* found that quality is lacking in Medicaid's care — and especially in the 60 percent of enrollees in managed care plans.[75] Here are a few of many examples where the level of care fell short:

- blood pressure control for hypertension control achieved: 58.4 percent for commercial plans, 53.5 percent for Medicaid
- timely prenatal care: 86.9 percent for commercial plans, 69.4 percent for Medicaid
- postpartum care: 77.2 percent for commercial plans, 40.7 percent for Medicaid
- recommended breast cancer screening: 75.1 percent for commercial plans, 52.6 percent for Medicaid
- glycated hemoglobin testing in diabetes patients: 82.6 percent for commercial plans, 73.4 percent for Medicaid
- glucose controlled in diabetes patients: 66.3 percent for commercial plans, 47.4 percent for Medicaid
- childhood immunization rate: 68.7 percent for commercial plans, 54.0 percent for Medicaid

In addition to these startling numbers, one must also focus on the hit that the elderly — and especially those in nursing homes — take from substandard Medicaid care. A study published in the *Journal of the*

75. Bruce E. Landon et al., "Quality of Care in Medicaid Managed Care and Commercial Health Plans," *Journal of the American Medical Association* 298, no. 14 (October 10, 2007).

*American Geriatrics Society* found, for instance, that "State Medicaid reimbursement rates appear to affect clinical decisions regarding the need for hospital admission and thresholds for nursing home use."[76] Mortality rates for those in nursing homes are also directly affected. Jennifer Troyer has found that the "overall mortality rate for Medicaid residents was 14.8% higher than the death rate for privately funded residents. When considering death within 1 year and 2 years, Medicaid residents' deaths were 4.2% and 7.8% higher, respectively."[77] She suggests that one possible reason for this is that Medicaid residents are segregated into lower-quality facilities — something that makes perfect sense in the context of dramatic attempts to cut costs.

Children also suffer from the lack of quality Medicaid care. For instance, Medicaid-covered children are more likely to receive care in institutions with higher mortality rates than their commercially insured counterparts. In addition, Medicaid recipients have higher death rates within groups of institutions that have similar overall mortality rates. Thus, even when Medicaid recipients are cared for at institutions demonstrating the lowest mortality, their overall odds of dying are more than twice that of commercial recipients.[78] Consider specifically, for instance, that in addition to poor children naturally having a higher risk of type 1 diabetes, they are significantly more likely to get substandard care as Medicaid enrollees. Low continuity of primary care for children on Medicaid contributed to disproportionately exacerbated conditions like diabetic ketocidosis.[79] And who could forget the February 2007 story of twelve-year-old Deamonte Driver's death from complications of an *infected tooth?* In addition to his Medicaid coverage having lapsed due to paperwork issues (it probably was mailed to a homeless shelter where his family was no longer staying), another difficulty was even finding a dentist to see in the first place. Though the federal government requires Medicaid programs to cover dental needs for children,

76. Orna Intrator, "Effect of State Medicaid Reimbursement Rates on Hospitalizations from Nursing Homes," *Journal of the American Geriatrics Society* 52 (2004): 1.

77. Jennifer L. Troyer, "Examining Differences in Death Rates for Medicaid and Non-Medicaid Nursing Home Residents," *Medical Care* 42 (2004): 1.

78. J. A. DeMone et al., "Risk of Death for Medicaid Recipients Undergoing Congenital Heart Surgery," *Pediatric Cardiology* 24, no. 2 (March 24, 2003): 101.

79. D. A. Christakis, "Continuity and Quality of Care for Children with Diabetes Who Are Covered by Medicaid," *Ambulatory Pediatrics* 1 (2001): 99.

the low Medicaid reimbursement rates reduce the number of dentists who will see such patients — particularly in rural areas.[80]

But we could also look at our imperiled newborns in a more narrow sense when using the triage analogy — in proportion to the good of the whole NICU patient population. Coming at it this way, in doing our proportional analysis of a particular NICU treatment we would compare the good of the treatment itself with the good it could do for all NICU babies in the particular state in question. So if Medicaid reimburses a hospital $467,567 for a 600-gram baby treated in the NICU, this is 467,567 fewer dollars to use for improving the fee ratio or for targeted eligibility expansion. And, as Gruber argues above, both would (1) significantly improve health outcomes for NICU babies (especially their mortality rates) and (2) significantly lower incidence of ELBW in the first place.

## Final Thoughts on the Medicaid-Triage Analogy

Recall John Lantos's quote from the introduction to this book: "Before the advent of neonatology, it was inconceivable to spend hundreds of thousands of dollars to save a baby's life. Today it has become routine and routinely disturbing."[81] Can we be so "routine" about how we spend these resources on Medicaid babies in the NICU?[82] The way we spend Medicaid dollars is, from the perspective of Catholic social teaching, something close to unconscionable. What do we say to those who get poor care on Medicaid due to poor reimbursement rates? What do we say to Janice Harris about her kidney stones or to Aaron England about his cancerous thyroid or to Jerry Springfield about his heart spasms? What do we say to Deamonte Driver's mother? How do we explain the millions of dollars we spend to save four imperiled newborn lives, while significantly less expensive (but often no less important) treatment is denied other needy patients?

We cannot explain it. The final section of the chapter makes two

80. See http://www.washingtonpost.com/wpdyn/content/article/2007/02/27/AR2007022702116.html (accessed August 21, 2010).

81. Lantos and Meadow, *Neonatal Bioethics*, 6.

82. The actual cost of NICU treatments — when factored over the person's lifetime — is dramatically higher than this.

kinds of arguments for how we should change our attitudes and practices for treatment of imperiled newborns: first are some general reforms, and second are reforms specific to Medicaid.

## General Reforms

Though the idea of limiting neonatal care in the interest of proportionate use of medical resources has barely reached the social consciousness of the United States (with the exception of Oregon), the central question asked in this book has been debated for some time now in Europe. In particular, the prestigious Nuffield Council on Bioethics in the U.K. put together a working party in 2005 to deal with thorny issues in neonatal treatment, and a central issue was resource distribution:

> The limitation of resources for healthcare is a major topic of debate in the UK, especially where the lives of babies are at stake. There is now much broader public awareness of the need for difficult choices to be made by the providers of national healthcare. We have discussed the difficult economic issues which have to be managed in neonatal medicine because more babies are able to survive than in the past. . . . Consequently, this has caused questioning of whether funds spent on resuscitating or prolonging the life of babies where the prognosis is very poor are spent appropriately.[83]

As we saw above with Medicaid, the council notes that comprehensive coverage of NICU treatment may not be possible "without cuts to other services so that, for example, spending more on the very young may reduce the amount available to help the elderly."[84] In the United

83. Nuffield Council on Bioethics, "Critical Care Decisions," 164. Interestingly, the next question the council asks is, "Can this be reconciled with the aim of healthcare professionals to 'treat the baby in front of them'?" If one accepts that relational anthropology of Catholic social teaching and of a physician's duty to treat the whole person — as was argued for in chapter 3 — then the answer to this question is yes.

84. Nuffield Council on Bioethics, "Critical Care Decisions," 164. Recall that in the introduction to this book we saw a specific example of this kind of consideration being taken very seriously by the U.K.'s national health service. Indeed, when the physician told the poor woman that "it was against the rules" to have her premature baby, the

States, however, we are far less likely to even consider, much less make, such difficult choices. Indeed, a 2007 study of physician preferences about resuscitation in the "gray zone" of viability found that "neonatologists place great emphasis on patient-orientated outcome variables (futility, viability, and morbidity), deemphasizing societal or personal concerns (resources, religion, and lawsuits)."[85] But if the central argument of this book is correct, the United States had better take a cue from the Nuffield Council and start looking at making some difficult decisions in the interest of proportionate use of health care resources. What follows are two sets of arguments and suggestions in this regard.

*Make illegal the using of resources for treatment of imperiled newborns that cannot possibly benefit from the treatment.*[86] Millions of dollars are spent each year in the NICU on babies who cannot possibly benefit from the treatment.[87] These kinds of cases are the easiest of all, because invoking the social quality of life model is not even necessary to make the critique (treatment is not medically indicated even if one is looking at it from the individualistically narrow point of view) — though doing so certainly does strengthen the case. The fact that we send these kinds of resources right down the drain, especially in light of our health care crisis, is totally unacceptable and ought to be prohibited regardless of the source: Medicaid, private insurance, and even cash.

Steve Leuthner has written extensively about what kinds of diagnoses and prognoses can, with certainty, be called "terminal."[88] In one group of terminal ailments we have both diagnostic and prognostic certainty:

trisomy 13, 15, or 18
triploidy

---

rules in question were set in place by the Nuffield Council; http://www.dailymail.co.uk/news/article-1211950/Premature-baby-left-die-doctors-mother-gives-birth-just-days-22-week-care-limit.html (accessed October 30, 2009).

85. Jaideep Singh, "Resuscitation in the 'Gray Zone' of Viability: Determining Physician Preferences and Predicting Infant Outcomes," *Pediatrics* 120 (2007): 523.

86. Perhaps it would be seen as, as Norm Fost calls it, a kind of neonatal "battery."

87. For instance, according to the Morbidity and Mortality Weekly Report (MMWR) cited earlier, on 290 terminal cases of anencephaly in 2003 we spent $1,090,270.

88. Steven R. Leuthner, *Fetal Palliative Care,* vol. 31 (Philadelphia: Elsevier, 2004), 649.

anencephaly/acrania
holoprosencephaly
large enecephaloceles
acardia
inoperable heart anomalies
severe clotting disorders
birth without pulmonary veins
Potter's syndrome/renal agenesis
multicystic/dysplastic kidneys
polycystic kidney disease

Another group, however, has prognostic certainty without diagnostic certainty:

thanatophoric dwarfism or lethal forms of ostenogenesis
    imperfecta
Potter's syndrome with unknown etiology
hydranencephaly
congenital severe hydrocephalus with absent or minimal brain
    growth

Though aggressive medical treatment should not be given — even at a parent's request or demand — forgoing such treatment does not constitute an abandoning of the child. Indeed, with proper palliative care this is not abandonment but rather doing what it is clearly in her best interest — even conceived from an individualistically narrow point of view. Given that many of these diagnoses and prognoses can be made *in utero*, early delivery of the baby may be called for, especially under the following circumstances: there is a reasonably good chance the child will die before birth and a parent wants the chance to hold and cuddle the child before she dies; there are medical complications possibly associated with a normal birth; the constant moving of the baby reminds the mother of the child's impending death; persons who are not aware of the diagnosis/prognosis are asking about the coming birth of the baby; etc. In such cases — again, at the request of a parent — labor could be induced, or a caesarean section done, and palliative care could be administered.

One might anticipate two objections here. First, one could certainly press the idea of "reliable" diagnoses and prognoses. There is always straight-up human error to consider — should we really be making such dramatic and final conclusions in light of this reality? Even something as supposedly obvious as anencephaly has had its share of misdiagnoses. Second, even if we are sure about the diagnoses and prognoses, do we really want to do literally no aggressive treatment of such newborns? Today's terminal conditions become tomorrow's treatable ones because some *do* choose to aggressively treat.

These are certainly objections worthy of consideration. While taking into account human error becomes that much more important when life-and-death issues are at stake, it is not something that is avoidable — and certainly not unique to the NICU. Individuals and families (and, indeed, some physicians) must make similarly dramatic decisions in other intensive care situations for older persons. Given human error, which can be substantial in this context,[89] there is virtually no case that one can predict with literally 100 percent certainty, but one could still accept as terminal cases where the accuracy *approaches* 100 percent. Indeed, one often finds that "human error" has an easily correctable cause: many of the more widely discussed misdiagnoses of anencephaly, for instance, were the result of deliberately shoddy work in order to make such babies available for cardiac donation.[90] About the second objection, it seems that in certain cases where advances in disease treatment are foreseeable, a separate legal route for clinical trials is needed. Such cases should have a funding path separate from Medicaid, private insurance, or private cash from the family of the baby. Rather, treatment should be funded just like any other clinical trial (perhaps by the National Institutes of Health or other like body) and should have the normal institutional review board oversight.

*Take significant steps to limit the "culture of overtreatment" in the NICU.* The NICU is perhaps one of the best places on earth to see a problematic "idolization" of biological life. It's also where one can see quite clearly humanity's problematic refusal to accept its own finitude and that of its resources. Several reforms need to take place.

*1. Merge Medicaid reimbursement rates in the NICU with other kinds of re-*

---

89. Geoffrey Miller, *Extreme Prematurity: Practices, Bioethics, and the Law* (Cambridge and New York: Cambridge University Press, 2007), 23.

90. AMA Council on Ethical and Judicial Affairs, "The Use of Anencephalic Neonates as Organ Donors," *Journal of the American Medical Association* 273 (1995): 1614-18.

*imbursement.* Although it certainly depends on the socioeconomic area
the hospital is in, NICUs generally have a high percentage of patients
funded by Medicaid. The rate usually varies between 50 and 80 percent
of a given census, with the average number[91] of babies on Medicaid being about 65 percent. Starting in the 1980s after Baby Doe, and continuing today, Medicaid reimburses for NICU care at a significantly
higher rate than it does for other kinds of care. Especially when one
considers the connection between public and private insurance (specifically, the latter generally taking the lead from the former), it is important that Medicaid not reimburse at a higher rate for NICU treatment
than for other kinds of treatment.

2. *Legal reform and education.* At times neonatal clinicians — especially after the Baby Doe case — were unclear about what the law was
and how it would be enforced. Laws supporting the culture of
overtreatment in the NICU (whether federal or state) need to be re-
pealed and an educational campaign started to make both clinicians
and hospital attorneys aware of the legal realities.

3. *Regulate new NICU building and expansion.* The dramatic move toward building of new NICUs since the late 1970s certainly has contributed to a culture of overtreatment. Lantos suggests that "From a public
policy perspective, the solution to this problem of the over-supply is
straightforward; stronger regulation could eliminate smaller NICUs or
at least make it less profitable for a small hospital to build and operate
a NICU."[92] Profitability would have already been reduced by the reforms made above, but an additional safeguard could be that, perhaps,
a certain number of NICU beds could only be built relative to a given
population.

4. *Change Medicaid requirements to reflect a proportionate distribution of
resources.* This will not only better distribute resources within Medicaid,
but because they use Medicaid rates as a baseline, it will also help spur
reform of how private insurers reimburse for neonatal care. Of course,
it is one thing to show that resources are disproportionately distributed within Medicaid, but it is quite another to make an argument for

91. This is about the average for the NICU at Memorial Hospital in South Bend, In-
diana. In an interview with the head neonatalogist there, Dr. Robert White, I discovered
that this generally reflects the average of the country as a whole.

92. Lantos and Meadow, *Neonatal Bioethics,* 134.

what a proportionate distribution might look like. Happily, we can look to some models that already exist for guidance and insight.

## The Oregon Model

During the 1980s the United States had a crisis with Medicaid similar to today's. Even then, Medicaid spending had

> increased dramatically and the program consumed a growing share of state budgets. In response, many states lowered eligibility standards for Medicaid to an income level well below the federal poverty line (FPL) and cut coverage for optional enrollee categories such as the medically needy. By the end of the decade, the health insurance program for poor Americans covered only 42 percent of the poor; in order to qualify for Medicaid, AFDC [Aid to Families with Dependent Children] recipients typically needed to live on incomes that were only 50 percent of the FPL. . . . In addition, those who were not "categorically eligible," such as low-income adults without children, were excluded from Medicaid in most states.[93]

Oregon bucked this trend in 1989 by passing the Oregon Basic Health Services Act. Instead of ratcheting down coverage based on eligibility, "Oregon proposed to extend Medicaid coverage to all persons living below the poverty line, regardless of traditional eligibility categories." Put simply, "Oregon said it intended to pay for enlarged Medicaid enrollment by covering fewer services."[94] If there was a budget shortfall, the state legislature could not cut eligibility to Medicaid, but rather had to ration care for those that were eligible. Essentially, a certain number of treatments would be covered by Oregon's Medicaid program, and the rest would not. But determining how to create such a list, as one might imagine, turned out to be a tricky business.

In creating the initial list, Oregon created a "health services commission" that used cost-effectiveness as its primary consideration —

93. Lawrence Jacobs, "The Oregon Health Plan and the Political Paradox of Rationing: What Advocates and Critics Have Claimed and What Oregon Did," *Journal of Health Policy, Politics and Law* 24 (1999): 163.

94. Jacobs, "The Oregon Health Plan," 163-64.

such that even very beneficial treatments might be rejected if the costs were high or only a few people could benefit from them. The commission did a cost-effectiveness analysis of over 1,600 health services but ended up with a list that was highly counterintuitive. For instance, office visits for thumb sucking were covered but lifesaving surgeries — such as appendectomies — were not. At least in part due to negative public reaction to the list, but also due to negotiations with federal authorities who needed to approve federal funding assistance, the commission abandoned cost-effectiveness as the primary consideration and made a new list. Cost was still a factor, but other factors took more priority, including benefit to the patient, benefit to society, and degree of "necessity." Intuition also played a significant factor as, even after the list was created, commissioners moved treatments "by hand" when seemingly very important services ended up low on the list.[95]

The program was formally implemented in Oregon in 1994, and the eligible population grew dramatically: from 10,000 in March 1994 to nearly 100,000 by December 1994 — far exceeding expectations. Because of these numbers, the state budget could not remain solvent without cutting treatments that everyone agreed counted as a "decent minimum" of coverage. And so, even though this was exactly what Oregon wanted to avoid, eligibility had to be cut anyway: assets tests were initiated and all full-time students were eliminated. To add insult to injury, cost cutting also included removing coverage for many procedures, including incapacitating hernias, tonsillectomies, and adenoidectomies.[96]

Interestingly, during the first stage of commission deliberations — the one that focused on cost-effectiveness — the very last two lines on its list referred to extremely low-birth-weight babies (under twenty-three weeks gestation or under 500 grams) and anencephalic babies.[97] This meant they were well beyond services likely to be treated. Indeed, the Oregon state legislature initially approved the list and then "approved funding up to and including line 587, leaving life support for ELBW babies and anencephalic babies (lines 708 and 709) well beyond

95. David C. Hadorn, "The Oregon Priority-Setting Exercise: Quality of Life and Public Policy," *Hastings Center Report* 21 (1991): 11-12.

96. Tom L. Beauchamp and James F. Childress, *Principles of Biomedical Ethics,* 5th ed. (New York: Oxford University Press, 2001), 256.

97. Mark J. Merkens and Michael J. Garland, "The Oregon Health Plan and the Ethics of Care for Marginally Viable Newborns," *Journal of Clinical Ethics* 12 (Fall 2001): 266-73.

the funding limit. If this list had been implemented, parents of such babies would have been confronted with the fact that Medicaid would not pay for life-supporting services for their infants."[98] However, when the second list came out, these life-supporting services no longer existed on their own — but rather as parts of more general kinds of treatments for newborns, including "life support for neuromuscular dysfunctions." Such treatments were high enough on the list to be funded.[99] But let us suppose that the dramatic move away from cost-effectiveness in the second list was a mistake. Let us consider that, perhaps, one way to proportionately distribute resources within Medicaid — especially for treatment of imperiled newborns — would be to create a similar list with disproportionate NICU treatments toward the bottom. Perhaps federal authorities could mandate that, to receive federal funds for Medicaid support (without which virtually no state Medicaid program could function), each state must create just such a list.

But there are good reasons to reject a model like Oregon's, which uses a list of "generic health states." To get a list that was manageable, the commission was forced to describe such states very broadly. For example, experiencing "trouble talking" incorporated everything from a slight lisp to being totally mute. All stages of esophageal stricture were placed in one category despite degrees of stricture varying widely in severity and cost. The same was true of renal failure and a host of other diseases. Anyone attempting to come up with a similarly manageable list today would be faced with the same problem. Interestingly, the issue with this model is similar to the "medical indications" model considered in chapter 2. In both cases the disease is unhelpfully abstracted from the broadly considered medical benefit, or best interests, of the patient. Beauchamp and Childress also bring to our attention the financial problems that need to be highlighted when considering such a model: "A basic question has haunted the Oregon Plan: How high can the cutoff line be set and still constitute a decent minimum package in accordance with the demands of social justice? The history of the plan demonstrates that the priority list may be an inadequate way to manage budget shortfalls, which have occurred in every year."[100]

---

98. Merkens and Garland, "The Oregon Health Plan," 266.
99. Merkens and Garland, "The Oregon Health Plan," 268.
100. Beauchamp and Childress, *Principles of Biomedical Ethics,* 257.

Still, there are positive things to highlight about the plan. It makes an honest effort to balance the severe tension between trying to provide (as Catholic teaching demands) a "decent minimum" of health services to the most vulnerable members of our society and controlling costs (even by considering refusal to cover treatment of ELBW babies) such that the state budget can remain solvent. It acknowledges the reality that we are rationing resources already and attempts to find a rational and morally defensible basis for doing so. As Paul Schotsmans points out, our culture needs to be more critical about the "hidden" priorities in the status quo of our health care system. The value of the Oregon plan was the promotion of public concern for, and participation in, public policy-making procedures in this regard. It is therefore necessary that a more systematic study be done on medical treatments and their various outcomes — and that the relevant health care data become public. Both information and policy transparency will help make people more alert and help them discuss on a more open level the priorities of various health care systems.[101] With these strengths of the Oregon plan in mind, let us consider another model for proportionately distributing resources within Medicaid.

## The Quality-Adjusted Life-Year

Rather than looking at a list of generic health states, perhaps we should evaluate more specific and individual treatments as a basis for controlling costs. One way to do this is to use something called the "quality-adjusted life-year" (QALY) — a concept devised by health economists to assess the relative cost-effectiveness of different treatments. Eric Matthews explains the basics quite well:

> The idea is that we can judge different treatments in terms of the number of years of extra life enjoyed by a successfully treated patient, multiplied by the quality of each of those years, as measured on a scale from 0 to 1. Thus, if a treated patient has 10 more years of life, each of which measured 0.5 on the quality scale, that treatment would have generated 5 QALYs. We can arrive at a "cost per QALY"

101. Engelhardt and Cherry, *Allocating Scarce Medical Resources*, 133.

for that treatment: suppose the treatment cost £1500, then the cost per QALY would be £300. Finally, we can compare this treatment with others in terms of their relative cost per QALY: if another treatment cost only £1000, but generated only 2 QALYs, then its cost per QALY, at £500, would be greater than that of the first treatment. It would be less cost-effective.[102]

With the QALY, then, we have an attempt to balance two aspects of the good of health care: its capacity for both life extension and life enhancement. The assumption here is that the trade-off between quantity and quality is accounted for in the multiplication of the two numbers. And, in fact, these kinds of trade-offs are balanced every day in medical decision making.

But determining the trade-off between quantity and quality is one thing — determining the "quality index" of a certain treatment in the first place is something else. What those who favor this approach do, especially in a macro-allocation context, "is take a checklist of factors that are likely to affect the perceived quality of life of normal people, and assign weightings to them . . . [and] the factors and their associated weightings are mostly so chosen as to reflect the feelings and considered judgments which the average or representative patient is likely to evince in practice, when faced with various forms of disability or discomfort, either in prospect or, better, having actually experienced them."[103]

Some might think this would discriminate wrongfully against those with a disability that brings about a low quality of life. But as Paul Menzel points out, this is not necessarily the case and "a common misperception." Medical treatments that do not save lives, but improve a low quality of life, "get more weight in any competition with lifesaving measures than they otherwise would have."[104] Consider a patient with renal failure and a quality of life index of 0.6. If dialysis treatment would give her ten years of life, at the cost of $30,000/year, the resulting $50,000/QALY price tag would undoubtedly place her treatment in

102. Eric Matthews and Michael Menlowe, *Philosophy and Health Care*, Avebury Series in Philosophy (Aldershot, England, and Brookfield, Vt.: Avebury, 1992), 40.

103. Helga Kuhse and Peter Singer, *Bioethics: An Anthology*, 2nd ed., Blackwell Philosophy Anthologies, vol. 25 (Malden, Mass., and Oxford: Blackwell, 2006), 453.

104. Matthews and Menlowe, *Philosophy and Health Care*, 65.

a relatively low priority position for rationing. In this case, having a low quality of life hurt the patient in the QALY rationing system. But consider another scenario where, instead of dialysis, her caregivers are considering a kidney transplant, which would raise her quality of life from 0.6 to 0.8 for ten years — producing 2.0 QALYs beyond dialysis. Let's say the transplant plus the subsequent treatments cost $60,000. Her roughly $30,000/QALY gain "puts her claim for a transplant in better stead against other services than if we ignored her jump in QOL."[105]

The main advantage of the QALY over the Oregon generic list of health states is that it allows for a more complete picture of the context to be considered. One part of that picture certainly is life-years added — something the Oregon system could not directly take into account for individuals. In addition, instead of having to decide whether or not to treat *anyone* with renal failure, Medicaid funds could be more nimbly allocated where they do the most good with respect to quality of life. One could refuse dialysis to a Medicaid enrollee who happens to be in a persistent vegetative state (where the quality of life index is zero or even negative) but offer dialysis to other patients who, though they might live just as long, would have a greater quality of life. Medicaid, after thorough research, could come up with a threshold of "dollars-per-QALY added." Treatments under that threshold would be covered, but treatments over it would not. This would have particular reference to the NICU, where treatments are very expensive and often have questionable length and quality of life outcomes.

However, though an improvement over the Oregon system, at least two important problems with the QALY make it a questionable model: (1) problems with balancing length of life and quality of life and (2) problems with determining and measuring quality of life.[106] On the former, David Hadorn points out that the QALY method "assumes that people see no difference between, say, one year of normal-quality life and ten years of life at one-tenth quality (whatever *that* is). The QALY approach assumes that a short, good life is of equal value to a long, ailing one. This assumption seems unlikely to be valid."[107] In-

---

105. Matthews and Menlowe, *Philosophy and Health Care*, 65.

106. Another problem is one of calculation and data gathering. But because this problem will also be associated with the ultimate argument, it will not be dealt with here.

107. Thomas A. Shannon, ed., *Bioethics*, 4th ed. (Mahwah, N.J.: Paulist, 1993), 424.

deed, the relationship between the value of quantity and quality of life seems far more complicated than simply multiplying quantity by a quality index of some kind.

But the latter problem is simply determining quality of life to begin with. As Hadorn asks, what does it even *mean* to speak of someone with a 0.1 quality of life index? How can we "quantify a *quality*, especially one so amorphous and ill-defined as quality of life"?[108] Furthermore, how could we possibly compare quality of life for one individual with that of another? Matthews, for instance, asks how we can "precisely compare the moral worth of saving the life of a heart patient by means of transplant surgery with that of enhancing the mobility of an old person by means of a hip replacement. How can we even place these two things on the same scales? Any comparisons between them must be based on qualitative judgments, not on simple mechanical conceptions of cost-effectiveness."[109] In addition, such judgments are almost totally subjective — with different answers given by healthy persons compared to those with disabilities. Indeed, a person with sight might consider blindness to significantly lower quality of life, whereas a blind person often does not share this judgment.[110]

In addition, QALYs suffer from a limitation shared by the Oregon generic health-states: limitation based on manageability. Recall that Oregon's system could not get as specific with diseases as it should have because it needed a list that was practically manageable. The QALY needs to define quality of life in a similarly limited way — usually with appeals to "disability and distress"[111] — and for the same practical reasons. But quality of life is often dependent on many factors that practical models are incapable of capturing. Michael Lockwood points out that quality of life includes at least the following: where one lives, one's social circumstances, what sort of job one has (if any), living alone or with a family, one's temperament and psychological makeup, the character of one's relationships with others, the authenticity of one's ac-

108. Shannon, *Bioethics,* 425.

109. Matthews and Menlowe, *Philosophy and Health Care,* 42.

110. The most striking evidence of this is the recent controversy over blind or deaf parents choosing embryos to be implanted who are also likely to be blind or deaf. They claim that their quality of life, far from being low, is actually a very rich (and perhaps even richer) kind of existence.

111. Matthews and Menlowe, *Philosophy and Health Care,* 57.

tions compared to one's principles, a sense of security and being in command of one's life, freedom to pursue life projects, degree of stress or boredom or frustration, sense of satisfaction and fulfillment in day-to-day living, and many, many other things the sum of which cannot possibly be captured by any kind of practical quantitative model.[112]

A final problem with defining quality of life in a medical treatment context is that many treatments that can be offered in clinics and by health care providers can improve quality of life but do not minister to *medical need* at all. Cosmetic surgery, for instance, could certainly improve one's quality of life — especially if one's employment or social status was largely based on one's physical appearance. Lockwood suggests, for instance, that (depending on the circumstances) a face-lift or hair transplant might produce more QALYs per unit cost than a hip replacement operation. But "would anyone really think that was sufficient reason for switching resources from hip replacements towards such cosmetic surgery? Surely not."[113]

QALYs, then, have too many problems to be accepted in their entirety as a model for proportionately distributing health care resources within Medicaid. However, as with Oregon, we can take away positive lessons from their consideration. One basic lesson is that we need to see treatments in a more individual and specific context — not just with regard to a generic treatment or disease/health state. Though it certainly seems that coming up with a quality of life index is perhaps hopelessly complex and problematic, and I am at pains to avoid its playing a role in this book's argument, it does not follow that we ought to completely abandon quality of life considerations altogether. Indeed, recall the original example of the kidney dialysis machine being used on the PVS patient and the non-PVS patient. Is there a way to capture the intuitively obvious case to be made that resources should be used on the latter patient rather than the former? Perhaps instead of using a vague and broad concept like quality of life we instead use a concept like relational capacity. Using this more narrow concept in determining which patient to treat would give us the intuitive result without forcing us to justify other, much more difficult, quality of life judgments.[114] Also, *length* of

112. Kuhse and Singer, *Bioethics*, 456.
113. Kuhse and Singer, *Bioethics*, 458.
114. More will follow on how this would work practically.

life does seem to be a legitimate factor to consider when making decisions on proportional distribution of resources and ought to be an aspect of QALYs used in Medicaid distribution.

## Why Pick on the NICU?

The context for the central argument of this book is the treatment of imperiled newborns in the NICU. However, especially if one accepts the length of life criteria of the QALY model in a cost-benefit analysis, one might argue that the proportionate distribution critique ought not to be brought first — or even at all — to the NICU. Consider first the actual dollars that might be saved by limiting such treatment. While the figures cited earlier in the chapter might seem high in the abstract, when compared to the total NICU expenses they are relatively small. In 1998 *Pediatrics* published a study conducted by Jeffery Stolz and Marie McCormick in which they found that "Policies denying care to infants born at 500, 600, or 700 g would lead to a total NICU care savings of 0.8%, 3.2%, and 10.3%, respectively." When applying the local survival rates for such birth weights, it would mean the death of "136, 575, and 2689 potential survivors annually."[115] The money saved seems relatively small compared to the lives that would be lost.

In addition, when one sees the expenses in the context of a comparison with other ICUs, treatment of imperiled newborns looks to be an even better bet. John Lantos and William Meadow have led studies and something bordering on a public campaign to show precisely this. In a 1993 study comparing costs and outcomes in the neonatal and medical ICUs (MICUs) — with respect to imperiled newborns and elderly patients — they found that "To the extent that allocation decisions are driven by concerns about distributive justice and the efficient use of scarce resources, it would be more justifiable to ration intensive care for the very old than the very young."[116] Their rationale was based on the following. NICU babies were more likely to die early and then have

115. Jeffery Stolz and Marie McCormick, "Restricting Access to Neonatal Intensive Care: Effect on Mortality and Economic Savings," *Pediatrics* 101 (1998): 344.

116. John Lantos and William Meadow, "Resource Allocation in Neonatal and Medical ICUs: Epidemiology and Rationing at the Extremes of Life," *American Journal of Respiratory Critical Care Medicine* 156 (1997): 185.

their chances of survival improve with each passing day. But precisely the opposite trend occurred with the elderly in the MICU, in which the population was increasingly likely to die the longer they stayed. Because imperiled newborns tend to die quickly, "most of the bed-days in the NICU are devoted to patients who ultimately survive. Because adults who die tend to have more prolonged courses in the ICU before succumbing, a much higher percentage of ICU bed-days are allocated to patients who ultimately die."[117] They suggest that proportionate resource distribution discussion "might be better framed in terms of number of ICU bed-days (a proxy for dollars) utilized by survivors (or nonsurvivors) divided by the total number of ICU patients bed-days/dollars expended." The conclusion being that "although survival for infants of extremely low birth weight may be very unlikely, the cost to society for the care of nonsurvivors is relatively low."[118] This is especially true when one thinks about the number of life-years added in the NICU versus the MICU.

Neonatal care has changed since 1993, however. Technology has improved such that even more lives are saved at the earliest stages of viability, but this also means that imperiled newborns who die take longer to do so. In a study conducted on imperiled newborns from 1991 through 2001, Lantos and Meadow found "a steady rise in the medical length of survival for doomed infants of approximately one-half day per year, from a median DOL [days of life] 2 to DOL 10. The average LOS [length of stay] for nonsurvivors paralleled this trend, rising from 5 to 17 days over the study period."[119] If true, this calls their original argument — that the vast majority of NICU bed-days are devoted to NICU survivors — into serious question. However, Meadow and Lantos believe that their argument still stands because, during the same time period, *overall survival* for imperiled newborns improved. This trend balanced the other such that "Nonsurvivors occupied a constant (and extremely small) fraction of NICU bed-days (% in every year and 7% for the decade overall)."[120] This paved the way for them to reiterate their

117. Lantos and Meadow, "Resource Allocation," 186.

118. Lantos and Meadow, "Resource Allocation," 187.

119. John Lantos and William Meadow, "Changes in Mortality for Extremely Low Birth Weight Infants in the 1990s: Implications for Treatment Decisions and Resource Use," *Pediatrics* 113 (2004): 1226.

120. Lantos and Meadow, "Changes in Mortality," 1228-29.

central claim from the previous article — one that challenges the fundamental position of this book:

> Several ethical consequences emerge from these observations. For infants with BWs 1000 g, BW-specific survival is so good that there are no ethically supportable claims for nonsupport as a function of either likelihood of death or of excess cost based on BW alone. Over the past decade, BW-specific survival for infants with BWs of 800 to 1000 g has improved to the point at which the same ethical rubric probably applies. For the tiniest ELBW infants (BW 450 to 600 g) considered at the time of their birth, they remain unlikely to survive. However, because at least half of these nonsurvivors will expire within 10 days, survival for the population of these infants who reach DOL 10 increases to at least 70% [which makes the treatment quite cost-effective].[121]

If Meadow and Lantos are correct, then the central focus of this book — with its particular emphasis on treatment of imperiled newborns — is wrongheaded. However, there are good reasons to doubt that "there are no ethically supportable claims" for restricting neonatal care in the interests of proportionate distribution of resources — based, at least in part, on complications and medical costs resulting from low birth weight.

Let's start with short-term costs. It isn't clear why one should think that bed-days with respect to survivors/nonsurvivors would be the best way to evaluate costs and benefits of ICU treatment. Why not use actual dollars spent? And even if that yielded a similar result (and Susan Schmitt's previously cited California study suggests it wouldn't), one would still need to properly account for Lantos's own point about various indirect costs: including contributing to a culture of overtreatment in the NICU that peels off needed dollars from other, more neglected areas of medicine. Also with regard to short-term costs, why should we think a savings of 14.3 percent of the NICU budget is not significant — and, if redistributed to other areas of Medicaid, not a more proportionate use of resources? Using Lantos's 2004 estimated figures as a baseline, let's conservatively estimate that total NICU expenditures was $26 billion in 2009. Giving comfort care to ELBW ba-

---

121. Lantos and Meadow, "Changes in Mortality," 1229.

bies below 700 grams would still produce a substantial savings of $3,718,000,000 per year.

But even if one were to dismiss the response made above to the short-term NICU costs and benefits (and there is good reason not to), the most powerful response to Lantos and Meadow is to point out that Medicaid dollars and other community resources spent on imperiled newborns are almost never limited to what is spent in the NICU. As the Nuffield Council points out, "Economic studies of premature birth and low birthweight have tended to overlook the costs, for example, of day-care services and respite care, as well as those borne by the local authorities, voluntary organizations and by families as a result of modifications of their everyday activities."[122] Though they should be considered in other contexts, let us ignore for now the very significant costs to families and private charities that future treatment and education of the imperiled newborn entail. Let us consider only costs borne by the community — since this is what we are after with regard to Medicaid in this section. If a baby is born in the NICU and funded by Medicaid, the follow-up physician and hospital visits, in-home nursing care, etc., will more than likely be paid for by Medicaid as well. Specialty education, if necessary, is also paid for by the community. All these *future* costs to the community must be taken into consideration in any true proportional analysis of how Medicaid monies are spent in the NICU.

A study published in the *Journal of the American Medical Association* found that infants of extremely low birth weight (less than 1,000 grams) are disproportionately likely to have considerable long-term health and educational needs.[123] Indeed, "ELBW children have extremely high rates of chronic conditions compared with NBW [normal birth weight] children. These conditions include asthma, cerebral palsy, and visual disability, as well as poorer cognitive ability, academic achievement, motor skills, and social adaptive functioning."[124] Predictably, ELBW babies had a significantly greater need for "services above routine" than children who were NBW. These included "visiting a physician regularly for a chronic condition, nursing care/medical proce-

122. Nuffield Council on Bioethics, "Critical Care Decisions," 122.

123. Maureen Hack, "Chronic Conditions, Functional Limitations, and Special Health Care Needs of School-Aged Children Born with Extremely Low-Birth-Weight in the 1990s," *Journal of the American Medical Association* 294 (2005): 318.

124. Hack, "Chronic Conditions," 323.

dures, occupational or physical therapy, special school arrangements, or an individualized education program. . . . Many children saw multiple specialists."[125]

It is notoriously difficult to estimate the costs of these treatments and services over time, but the Nuffield Council cited an EPICure study that looked at spending (in pounds) over twelve months at age six and compared the cost of ELBW children versus a control group born at full term. Here are the results in British pounds:[126]

| Cost Category | Cost for ELBW | Cost for Full-Term Child |
|---|---|---|
| Hospital Inpatient | 605 | 116 |
| Hospital Outpatient | 255 | 53 |
| Community Health | 422 | 104 |
| Drug Cost | 10 | 3 |
| Education | 7,620 | 3,470 |
| Additional Family Expenses | 573 | 120 |
| Indirect Costs | 56 | 17 |

These numbers are dramatic enough, but they are even more striking when considered over the entire life of the patient. Consider "Baby Sidney," the subject of the important *HCA v. Miller* case in Houston, Texas, in 1998. Sidney's parents, under advice from their physician, decided they would not resuscitate her after she was born, and there was an official order made to not have a neonatalogist present at the time of her birth. However, hospital officials told Sidney's father, Mark Miller, that hospital policy required that Sidney be resuscitated without consent. Sidney was born, resuscitated, and left so physically and neurologically devastated that she has never been able to walk, talk, or feed herself.[127] This is relevant to this book not so much because of the decision to give aggressive treatment, but because of what happened after the jury found the hospital guilty and forced it to pay the Miller family compensatory damages for Sidney's medical expenses. The jury found:

125. Hack, "Chronic Conditions," 323.

126. Nuffield Council on Bioethics, "Critical Care Decisions," 85.

127. Report of the Court of Appeals for the Fourteenth Court of Appeals District in Texas in *HCA, INC. v. Sidney Ainsley Miller,* 4-10.

a. Reasonable expenses of necessary care for Sidney Miller in the past: $900,000.
b. Reasonable expenses of necessary medical care that, in reasonable probability, Sidney Miller will incur in the future: $28,500,000.

The hospital's own expert witness even testified to the expense of the procedures the jury used to calculate damages: pediatrician visits, neurosurgeon/neurologist visits, routine medical care, CAT scans, EEGs, emergency room visits, blood work, shunt surgery, shunt revisions, medications, physician/occupational/speech therapy, and others.[128]

The jury awarded the money to the Millers with the expectation that they would have to pay for the future medical expenses, but if Sidney had been on Medicaid her parents would have been unable to afford her care and the entire expense would have been borne by the community. When deciding about proportionate use of Medicaid resources in treating imperiled newborns, then, one cannot simply look at NICU costs in the abstract (though these numbers are dramatic in and of themselves); one must instead look at costs to Medicaid and the community over the lifetime of the patient. Far from there being "no ethically supportable claims" for giving comfort care to imperiled newborns based on resources, in light of our tragic health care and Medicaid crisis, it seems clear that a choice to treat a single NICU patient that will result in the spending of millions and millions of dollars over her lifetime is a disproportionate use of resources.

Though Meadow and Lantos overstep in claiming that NICU treatments are more cost-effective than other kinds of intensive care, a weaker claim that other kinds of medical care could be critiqued by the social quality of life model does in fact have merit. Though the specific factors to be considered in how to proportionately allocate resources would be different, there is no reason why one would have to in principle limit the social quality of life model to the context of neonatal treatment. Though it obviously goes beyond the scope of this book to suggest what this might look like, it is another direction for future study and work.

128. Report of the Court of Appeals, 37.

## Discrimination against the Disabled: Redux

In chapter 2 I attempted to show that the central argument being offered was not discrimination against the disabled. But if taking these kinds of long-term costs into consideration is the key move in showing why we should limit neonatal care rather than other kinds of care, then it does become difficult to see how the book could avoid the discrimination charge. Such long-term costs appear to be directly related to the disabilities of Baby Sidney and others like her. This seems to be exactly what one has in mind when one thinks about discrimination on the basis of disability.

In chapter 2 I maintained that there was nothing *necessarily* discriminatory about the social quality of life model as applied to imperiled newborns — even though disabled newborns will generally not fare as well as those without disabilities. Long-term costs of *any* kind could be taken into consideration — they do not *necessarily* need to be directly related to a disability. Again, consider the imperiled newborn with severe heart disease that will require constant surgeries and expensive medicine over the course of his life but will otherwise have no problems and lead a flourishing life. Such a person is not disabled but might be denied treatment under the social quality of life model as applied to imperiled newborns.

Perhaps a thought experiment will help drive the point home. Let us suppose a ferocious fire has broken out on the first floor of an understaffed rural hospital and one security guard has been given the task of clearing the second floor of patients because the fire department is quite far away. Suppose also that the floor has two wings: one wing has patients recovering from heart disease and the second wing has paraplegic patients currently in rehab. The security guard, in such a tragic situation where people are likely to die either way given the advanced stage of the fire, decides to go to the wing of those recovering from heart disease since they are able to walk on their own out of the hospital. In warning them of the danger and seeing them safely out he will save far more lives than if he went to the other wing and carried or wheeled each individual patient out of the hospital. Suppose that in doing so the security guard is unable to save the second-wing patients because by the time he is finished seeing the first-wing patients out the fire makes getting to the second wing impossible.

Could one justly complain that he engaged in wrongful discrimination against the disabled? Of course not. The fact that they were disabled was not the reason he chose to not save them first — rather, it was because it would take more resources (time) than he could have responsibly used in such a tragic situation. Indeed, if the second wing had had postcosmetic-surgery patients who were drugged such that he would also have had to wheel or carry them out of the hospital he would have made exactly the same kind of tragic calculation. In both hypothetical cases, discrimination on the basis of disability as such plays no role at all in his reasoning — only just distribution of his resources. The same is true of the social quality of life model with regard to imperiled newborns: discrimination as such never directly enters into consideration, but rather only indirectly as it (along with other factors) contributes to disproportionate use of resources.

## Proportionate Use of Medicaid Resources in the NICU: A Suggestive Proposal

Making specific policy proposals is dangerous territory for ethicists.[129] Our expertise concerns the values that should affect policy — others are often better in seeing the way forward and anticipating the unexpected twists and turns (and unintended consequences) that always accompany this part of the process. In addition, when deciding whether or not to treat an imperiled newborn on Medicaid in the NICU in light of the social quality of life model and Catholic social teaching, one must rely heavily on one's ability to predict outcomes: about survivability, about future disease and health, and about costs to treat such disease. If we cannot with relative accuracy predict whether or not a baby will survive, what kind of life the baby will have if she survives, and how much it will cost to treat and care for the baby both in the NICU and over her life, then we are left with too little information to make a judgment as final and as dramatic as withholding or withdrawing treatment from an imperiled newborn. The citation of Geoffrey Miller

---

129. Catholic social teaching is happily aware of this as well — and specifically acknowledges that its policy proposals do not carry the same weight as the values that undergird them.

above reminds us that prognostic mistakes are disturbingly common. Indeed, the Nuffield Council is just one of many players in this discussion who lament our current inability to make such predictions:

> Neonatal critical care decisions are particularly difficult because of the lack of information from long-term follow up on which to base predictions of future health outcomes. It is crucial that accurate and up-to-date evidence from research is available to doctors and parents about the risk to and likely outcomes for babies in whom a birth abnormality or genetic disorder has been recognized antenatally or in the newborn period, as for extremely premature babies. . . . Our view is that data linkage with longer-term events in later stages of a child's life, through adolescence to adulthood, captured through NHS health records and educational records, will provide crucial information on outcomes.[130]

Meadow and Lantos predict that "Accurate and timely prediction of persistent residual morbidity for NICU survivors looms as the next ethical frontier."[131] Until that frontier is explored in more detail, however, it is not prudent to make hard-and-fast recommendations about how to limit treatment of certain imperiled newborns with respect to Medicaid beyond what already has been said in this chapter. However, it is certainly prudent and important to make some broad suggestions about a practical model for limiting treatment, what factors should be taken into consideration in such a model, and what relative weight to give such factors. In addition, the model will help give researchers a sense of what kinds of studies are necessary to get the information needed.

A May 5, 2008, article in the *Boston Globe* reported that a task force of physicians from the Centers for Disease Control and Prevention, the Department of Homeland Security, and the Department of Health and Human Services came up with a "grimly specific" list of persons they believe should not be treated in a pandemic where medical resources are limited: people older than eighty-five, those with severe trauma, severely burned patients older than sixty, those with severe mental impairment, those with severe chronic disease, and others. They recommended that hospitals put together a triage team to prepare for such a

---

130. Nuffield Council on Bioethics, "Critical Care Decisions," 166.
131. Lantos and Meadow, "Changes in Mortality," 1229.

situation.[132] Though one may certainly object to some of the reasoning used to arrive at this list, the task force should be commended for attempting to prepare for the difficult decisions that must be made in a future triage situation. However, we are *already* in a triage situation with Medicaid, and an even stronger urgency should exist to think about Medicaid with the grim realism of the pandemic task force. Both to remind us of the gravity of this urgency and for ease of determining how to treat or not to treat certain imperiled newborns, perhaps such newborns at the time of their birth (and subsequently as evaluations/circumstances change and emerge) could be put into one of four medical triage categories. Here is a suggestive list:

> RED. "Must Treat." Data show that the baby should be given aggressive medical treatment. Unless diagnosed previously with a terminal disease, all babies for the first three days after birth will be in this category and given a chance to "declare themselves," since most babies who die do so in the first three days.
> YELLOW. "Unclear — Emergent." Data at this point make it unclear whether or not to treat the baby. However, the circumstances are such that a decision must be made quickly by the parent or guardian in consultation with clinicians. Here, perhaps, the Lantos-studied "clinical intuitions" of neonatal physicians and nurses would be given significant weight.
> GREEN. "Unclear — Nonemergent." Data at this point make it unclear whether or not to treat the baby. However, the circumstances are such that a decision need not be made quickly and can incorporate more study, the convention of an ethics consultation, longer and deeper conversations between family and clinicians, etc.
> BLACK. "Must Not Treat." Data show that the baby should be given palliative care.

An algorithm would need to be created into which one could feed data to produce one of these four categories.[133] Data would be of the following two kinds.

---

132. Lindsey Tanner, "Who Should MDs Let Die in a Pandemic?" *Boston Globe,* May 5, 2008.
133. Perhaps, though it would include more factors, it would mirror the algorithm

*Survivability and Length of Life Predictors.* Many variables would be factored into this group of data. Birth weight seems to be a key tool, but since babies are getting bigger, gestational age would probably play a larger role and should be weighted in the algorithm such that no baby under a certain gestational age should be treated. However, because the empirical data show that black babies and female babies do better than their white and male counterparts, race and gender should be factored in as well. Other things to consider: SNAP and APGAR scores, prenatal care and tests, maternal health and steroid use, and other data that clinicians would be better able to assess. The relative weight of each of these pieces of data should be a focus for future study.

*Short- and Long-Term Costs of Treatment.* Again, this data group would consider many variables. Of course, one would need the first data group to predict and estimate both short-term NICU treatment costs and costs for follow-up treatment over the life of the patient. One would then need to study in more depth the relationship between a certain level of premature birth and/or congenital disease and short/long-term costs for Medicaid. Emphasis should be given to studying this with regard to particularly common and expensive diseases. Obviously, total costs should be weighted in the algorithm such that the more costs a treatment produces the less likely it will be considered proportionate with the common good. But perhaps the weighting should go further. Building on Todd Whitmore's insight that Catholic social teaching on the universal destination of goods implies a "maximum living wage,"[134] perhaps we could talk about a "maximum medical benefit" (relative to total health care resources available, of course) that is justly available to a person from the community over the course of her lifetime. What that number would be needs to be the subject of further study and reflection, but perhaps a baseline figure could be relative to the cost of adding those to Medicaid who aren't quite impoverished enough to make the cut — like those mentioned previously who were dropped from TennCare.

---

used in the Tyson study to come up with a "predictor" (available for public online use) for imperiled newborn outcomes.

134. Todd David Whitmore, "Catholic Social Teaching: A Synthesis" (unpublished paper), 45.

Much would need to happen to make something like the above possible. Much research and study would be needed regarding predicting outcomes and estimating costs,[135] and also more study and thinking about the values behind the relative weights of certain kinds of data — and then about how to create an algorithm that reflects the values and weights. Obviously, this is a challenging project that would involve persons with different kinds of expertise: physicians, researchers, economists, statisticians, philosophers, theologians, etc. However, the fruits of such a project would be great in that instead of rationing Medicaid care in the haphazard and unjust way we are today, we would have a system in place that transparently and publicly attempted to find a morally defensible method of distributing medical resources in our society's tragic situation of medical want. But let me be absolutely clear: the previous section is merely meant to be suggestive. More information and reflection are needed before any hard-and-fast argument could be prudently made — to say nothing of actually enacting a public policy.

## A Preferential Option for the Poor?

Catholic social teaching "requires that the poor, the marginalized and in all cases those whose living conditions interfere with their proper growth should be the focus of particular concern. To this end, the preferential option for the poor should be reaffirmed with all its force." This is a "special form of primacy in the exercise of Christian charity" that embraces not only those who are considered traditionally poor (the hungry, needy, homeless, etc.) but also specifically "those without healthcare."[136] If these reforms are directed primarily at Medicaid, and Medicaid is the health insurance for the poor, then one might reasonably wonder how this book could possibly claim to be consistent with Catholic social teaching. My policy suggestions, far from a preferential option for the poor, sound like precisely the opposite. Could I possibly

135. Interestingly, we are on the verge of technology that may dramatically assist in this goal: complete genetic mapping at birth. This would make it "possible to identify the raised risk of developing an array of conditions"; http://www.timesonline.co.uk/tol/news/uk/science/article5689052.ece (accessed August 12, 2009).

136. Pontifical Council, *Compendium*, 86.

be arguing that if one is poor, then one will have NICU care curtailed —
but if one is wealthy enough to have one's own insurance, then we won't
regulate it at all? Furthermore, many of babies on Medicaid in the
NICU, especially in urban areas, are racial minorities. Is this book essentially arguing de facto that we should let poor, black babies die? If so, it
is hard to see how it could even be taken seriously as a piece of scholar-
ship — much less be congruent with the Catholic social tradition.

This is a powerful argument and one to which there must be an adequate response. I want to make three careful and respectful rejoinders.
First, does it follow that resources should not be distributed proportionally within a given group because that group has been wrongfully
discriminated against? Let us continue the analogy of the battlefield
triage situation. Suppose a black Civil War regiment had just finished
engaging the enemy in battle and a white triage medic, assigned to the
regiment, comes on the scene. Suppose also that the U.S. government
was complicit in wrongful discrimination by assigning only one medic
to the regiment when in fact it required three. The medic, despite the
larger injustice of discrimination against the regiment, should not *add*
to the injustice by refusing to proportionately distribute medical resources — even if other white regiments are not forced to make the
same tragic choices he has. If he passes over the first patient he sees because the soldier would take too long to stabilize relative to the needs
of the other soldiers for which he is responsible, he is not being racist.
He is making a decision based on the factors and variables over which
he has control and to which he has been assigned. Similarly, this chapter's argument about Medicaid does not presuppose control of how
health care resources are distributed more broadly, but only with regard to public policy about how community resources are spent. It is
true that it is a grave injustice that only one triage medic was assigned
to the black regiment — and it is true that it is a grave injustice that we
spend so little on Medicaid compared to the medical needs of the
poor.[137] However, neither is a legitimate excuse for disproportionately
distributing the resources that do exist.

137. Though it is the case that a disproportionate number of Medicaid babies are
black, and limitation of Medicaid NICU resources would disproportionately affect
blacks, it can hardly be said that the constructive proposal with regard to Medicaid is de
facto racist. This is because built into the algorithm, and based on studied medical outcomes, would be a significant (30-100 percent?) advantage of blacks over whites.

Second, there is indeed some regulation — both direct and indirect — of private insurance proposed in this chapter already. Direct regulation comes in the form of making it illegal to treat, and for insurance companies to cover with aggressive treatment, a host of terminal neonatal ailments. In addition, private spending on NICU care is indirectly regulated by attacking the culture that produces overtreatment — and thus overspending — in the first place.

Finally, private insurance companies often look to Medicaid for the "OK" to make policy and reimbursement changes. If Medicaid makes a change, then private insurance companies generally follow suit. This happened in physician billing, for instance. When Medicaid insisted that the attending physician actually be a part of a treatment in order for it to be billed (i.e., it was not just the work of a resident physician), all the private insurance companies immediately demanded the same thing. The connection is even more direct for reimbursement rates. Private insurance carriers often pay, particularly for treatment at out-of-network facilities, based on a percentage of something called the CMS Rate. The Center for Medicare and Medicaid Services determines its reimbursements for all medical services and publishes them annually,[138] thus allowing for private insurance to use their rates as a baseline. Most pay more, but if Medicaid were to lower its reimbursement rate for a given procedure, the private insurers would likely lower prices as well. What this means is that if the suggested Medicaid regulations of this chapter were enacted, it is more than likely that the reforms would be picked up by private insurers too — particularly if they were helped along with federal tax breaks for adopting the same system. After all, the short- and long-term costs of choosing to treat imperiled newborns covered by private insurance are also problematic for these companies — they drive up premiums for their members, hurt profits for their shareholders, etc. Once this change "cycles through," private insurance premiums would go down such that some of the poor who do not qualify for Medicaid could possibly afford private insurance. This would most certainly be a preferential option for the poor.

Catholic social teaching's critique of the attitudes and practices of treatment of imperiled newborns in the NICU found that they were

138. http://www.cms.hhs.gov/home/medicaid.asp (accessed June 23, 2008).

not consistent with a proportionate distribution of resources directed toward the common good: a decent minimum of health care for all. While a systematic discussion about wholesale changes to our health care system is beyond the scope of this book (though they will be gestured at in the conclusion), the reforms suggested in this chapter at least move us toward that goal. Resources would be freed up to either (1) improve physician and hospital reimbursement rates (thus improving care) or (2) expand the number of impoverished that can qualify for Medicaid — both of which would move many closer to having a decent minimum of health care. The latter would obviously do so by giving people health insurance who otherwise could not afford it (like, again, our TennCare examples), but the former would allow those on Medicaid to get needed care by seeing physicians they normally could not because of the low reimbursement rates.

But, importantly, we could even do this in a way that would not take our focus off of poor babies. My discussions with health care providers in several states have produced significant anecdotal evidence that providers of prenatal care, more and more, do not see Medicaid patients because of the very real fear they will lose money in the process. Many poor pregnant women, especially in rural areas, get care late or not at all. Improving Medicaid reimbursement rates in that area with targeted expansions, for example, would lower the incidence of ELBW births and start a cycle that would lessen the need for NICU care in the first place. Actual studies back up anecdotal evidence that Medicaid reform for prenatal care leads to better postnatal outcomes. UCLA researchers Janet Curie and Jeffrey Grogger, for instance, found that higher income cutoffs for Medicaid eligibility led to increased prenatal care use, which led to a small but significantly reduced risk of Medicaid mothers having very low-birth-weight babies.[139] Far from abandoning Medicaid babies, limiting NICU care in this way could actually *improve* overall care and outcomes for poor infants.

139. Janet Curie and Jeffrey Grogger, "Medicaid Expansions and Welfare Contractions: Offsetting Effects on Maternal Behavior and Infant Health," *Journal of Health Economics* 21 (2002): 313-35.

# Conclusion

*Do the sometimes staggering costs of neonatal intensive care mean that at some point the economics of care determine the meaning of best interests [of the infant]? We shy away from such considerations, and this is undoubtedly a healthy response. But how long we can sustain it I do not know.*

Richard McCormick[1]

This book has attempted to systematically consider some important facts that, when considered jointly in the same health care context, have dramatic implications. The health care system of the United States, at the time this book goes to press, leaves nearly 50 million of its people without health insurance of any kind and many millions more with insurance that does not meet their medical needs. (And, at best, many millions will still be left without coverage even if health care reform is enacted.) This is due to a number of complex factors, but perhaps the most important one is that we distribute resources, not with regard to patient population need, but with regard to considerations like profitability of treatment, ability of the patient to pay, political trends, the sympathetic or unsympathetic nature of the patient, the "culture" of certain areas of medicine, etc. Rationing of health care resources based on these criteria often results in disproportionate distri-

---

1. Richard A. McCormick, "The Best Interests of the Baby," *Second Opinion* 2 (July 1986): 21

bution and therefore unjust treatment — with certain patients getting huge shares of our medical resources and others getting dramatically smaller shares or even no share at all.

An important example of this disproportionality, this book has argued, is treatment of certain imperiled newborns in the neonatal intensive care unit (NICU). Especially when critiqued by the social quality of life model in light of Catholic social teaching, the "culture of overtreatment" in the NICU has been found to be in need of serious reform. This is not because imperiled newborns are less than full persons without a right to be considered on the same level as any other patient, but rather because what is in a newborn's best interest cannot be isolated from the duty of all to live in right relationship with the rest of humanity in conformity with the common good of all. Part of what it means to live in right relationship is to use only a proportionate amount of resources available in one's community. And given the dramatic numbers offered in chapter 4, it seems that some treatment of imperiled newborns is disproportionate with the common good. Such treatment, in light of the finitude of our resources (and of our human condition more generally), ought to be forgone.

Quite appropriately, many (including the author of this book) are very uncomfortable with such a conclusion. Such discomfort might tempt one to shy away from dealing with the reality of our tragic health care situation. However, as Duff and Campbell remind us, we cannot live outside the human condition — and this condition is riddled with tragedy. For if "we resist accepting tragedy as part of human experience, we fail too often to deal with tragedy, and thus we cannot discover and adopt the least tragic choice in situations where only tragic choices exist."[2] To simply let our health care resources be distributed the way they are currently — in a de facto triage situation — is a greater injustice than the remedy proposed in this book.

But as was mentioned in chapter 3, dealing with this tragic reality by forgoing treatment to imperiled newborns cannot be our only response to the problem. It is true that we will never fully eradicate disproportionate treatment in any health care system, but we can take further steps even beyond what this book argues. Not only can the critique of the so-

2. Fred M. Frohock, "Euthanasia and the Newborn: Conflicts regarding Saving Lives," *Ethics* 99, no. 3 (April 1989): 286.

cial quality of life model in light of Catholic social teaching be leveled at areas of medicine outside of the NICU, but we need not accept our current health care system's general structure as it now exists. Perhaps the most obvious example of "structural sin" in our culture is a health care system that causes the poor and the old — who are at high risk for disease already — to have dramatically worse health care than the financially comfortable and young. There is no need to take for granted this kind of system. Though it obviously goes beyond the scope of this book to make an argument in this regard, it is certainly worth mentioning some basic points about this in the conclusion and as a direction for further work.

Given the dominant political culture in this country, even as we have another national discussion about health care reform, it is highly unlikely that system-wide change that avoids the above problems will come in the foreseeable future. However, let us look again at one result of the Oregon debate over rationing:

> In Oregon, the rhetoric of rationing pulled into the open decisions that privately occur every day and that deny services to uninsured or underinsured Americans. OHP's [Oregon Health Plan] experience points to an unanticipated but possible political benefit of rationing rhetoric: it reconfigured debate toward openly acknowledging, as a society, what medical services Americans — even the politically eviscerated poor — should receive or go without. And it put politicians in the vulnerable position of pulling the plug on particular medical services. Paradoxically, a process ostensibly aimed at saying no might force voters and politicians — as it did in Oregon — to recoil in horror and say yes.[3]

In the short term, my hope is that we more proportionately allocate resources in the lower tier of the system, but the long-term hope is that many "recoil in horror" at the conclusion of this book and say yes to system-wide reform. Many citizens are aware of the plight of the uninsured and underinsured in the United States — and yet this is apparently not horrific enough to shift the political culture to say yes to dramatic and system-wide change that refuses to abandon several dozen

3. L. Jacobs, "The Oregon Health Plan and the Political Paradox of Rationing: What Advocates and Critics Have Claimed and What Oregon Did," *Journal of Health Policy, Politics and Law* 24 (1999): 178.

million persons. Though this is certainly not the central reason I made the argument I did, perhaps forgoing lifesaving treatment for babies in the NICU will be enough to give our culture the shock it needs to clear the conceptual space needed for this kind of systematic shift in thinking about health care.

What would such a system-wide shift look like? Again, it goes beyond the scope of this book to make an argument, but a broadly Roman Catholic understanding according to the National Conference of U.S. Catholic Bishops would require that the following criteria be met:[4]

- *Universal Access.* Whether it preserves and enhances the sanctity and dignity of human life from conception until natural death.
- *Priority Concern for the Poor.* Whether it gives special priority to meeting the most pressing health care needs of the poor and underserved, ensuring that they receive quality health services.
- *Comprehensive Benefits.* Whether it provides comprehensive benefits sufficient to maintain and promote good health, to provide preventive care, to treat disease, injury, and disability appropriately, and to care for persons who are chronically ill or dying.
- *Pluralism.* Whether it allows and encourages the involvement of public and private sectors, including the voluntary, religious, and nonprofit sectors, in the delivery of care and services; and whether it ensures respect for religious and ethical values in the delivery of health care for consumers and for individuals and institutional providers.
- *Quality.* Whether it promotes the development of processes and standards that will help to achieve quality and equity in health services, in the training of providers, and in the informed participation of consumers in decision making on health care.
- *Cost Containment and Controls.* Whether it creates effective cost-containment measures that reduce waste, inefficiency, and unnecessary care; measures that control rising costs of competition, commercialism, and administration; and measures that provide incentives to individuals and providers for effective and economical use of limited resources.
- *Equitable Financing.* Whether it ensures society's obligation to fi-

4. Kevin D. O'Rourke and Philip Boyle, *Medical Ethics: Sources of Catholic Teachings,* 3rd ed. (Washington, D.C.: Georgetown University Press, 1999), 181-82.

nance universal access to comprehensive health care in an equitable fashion, based on ability to pay; and whether proposed cost-sharing arrangements are designed to avoid creating barriers to effective care for the poor and vulnerable.

Though the Catholic Church admits that it is no expert in the creation or practical application of economic or health care systems that would most likely meet these criteria, it goes without saying that achieving this kind of reform is a tall order — especially in light of the hyper-autonomous culture of the United States. The Catholic Health Association has therefore argued that "While change is needed immediately, it is acknowledged that systemic change is most likely to be a gradual process, rather than occurring all at once."[5] A sequential strategy is needed to achieve the change required. But before our culture can start down this path with the urgency required to push through to the final goals, it is worth noting that the proper motivation and energy need to be present to shift our American values in this area. Again, perhaps nontreatment of certain imperiled newborns would serve as just such a needed motivation and energy creator.

But what do we do in the meantime? Suppose we do develop the technological capability for getting the predictive outcome data necessary for prudently limiting neonatal care such that it is in conformity with the common good: What about the Medicaid babies who don't get care? Do we simply sit back and let them die? Not if we are convinced by the example of the early Christians. Recall from chapter 1 that in the ancient Greco-Roman world

> by far the most common social reason for exposing a newborn was poverty. One more mouth to feed might all too easily mean taking food from family members who already suffered hunger. Indeed . . . it appears some families had genuine hope that their children would be saved — leaving the infant at a street corner, near a public building like a temple, or even at spots just outside a city or village that were specifically designed for exposure. Such hope was not always misplaced. Though scholars disagree as to the rates of survival, it appears that at least some of these infants became foster children and less fortunate

5. The Catholic Health Association of the United States, "Continuing the Commitment: A Pathway to Health Care Reform" (April, 2000), 9.

ones were picked up to be used as slaves or prostitutes. At any rate, the fact that this kind of exposure was common may say less about the attitude of the parents or culture toward the moral status of such infants than it does about the social realities with regard to scarcity of resources — and the desperation that such scarcity would drive some families who clearly wanted to give their infant child a chance at life.[6]

Early Christians saw it as their moral duty (even when subjected to ridicule by the surrounding culture) to save these infants who required a disproportionate amount of resources for their family to sustain. A similar situation would be the modern-day result if the central argument of this book informs our public policy with regard to treatment of imperiled newborns. Infants whose treatment would be forgone today would be analogous to infants exposed in the ancient world by families who could no longer afford their care, but would hope for their adoption after being exposed. Instead of nuclear families being unable to provide for them given a tragic lack of resources, our wider "social family" (considered, perhaps, as individual Medicaid programs — or a federal Medicaid program should we go in that direction) is unable to provide for them also because of a lack of resources — at least as our health care system is set up right now. Just as ancient Christians adopted these children at such a rate that it became an identifying mark of scorn and ridicule for their community, today's Christians would need to step up in a similar way. Hospitals — especially those with Roman Catholic affiliation — should set up charitable programs such that their NICUs could take certain babies who were denied treatment via Medicaid (perhaps those who were refused treatment primarily because of its short- and long-term expense) and fund their care. And anyone who is convinced by the example of the ancient Christians should then feel compelled to support such programs[7] financially through donations. And, if also convinced by Catholic social teaching, one should feel compelled to do so not simply by giving "from one's surplus" resources, but by sacrificing in a way similar to that of the early Christians: in a way that considers these infants as part of one's family. For, in light of Christian solidarity, that is exactly who they are.

6. O. M. Bakke, *When Children Became People: The Birth of Childhood in Early Christianity* (Minneapolis: Augsburg Fortress, 2005), 30.

7. As well as other programs and charities that would support the child's long-term needs.

# Bibliography

AMA Council on Ethical and Judicial Affairs. "The Use of Anencephalic Neonates as Organ Donors." *Journal of the American Medical Association* 273 (1995).

Arras, John D. "Toward an Ethic of Ambiguity." *Hastings Center Report* 14 (April 1984): 25-33.

Arras, John, and Nancy Rhoden. "Withholding Treatment from Baby Doe: From Discrimination to Child Abuse." *Milbank Memorial Fund Quarterly* 63 (Winter 1985): 18-51.

Beauchamp, Tom L., and James F. Childress. *Principles of Biomedical Ethics.* 5th ed. New York: Oxford University Press, 2001.

Benedict XVI. *Caritas in Veritate.* (2009).

Boyle, Joseph. "A Case for Sometimes Tube-Feeding Patients in Persistent Vegetative State." In *Euthanasia Examined: Ethical, Clinical, and Legal Perspectives,* edited by John Keown, 189-99. Cambridge: Cambridge University Press, 1995.

Camosy, Charles. "Common Ground on Surgical Abortion? — Engaging Peter Singer on the Moral Status of Potential Persons." *Journal of Medicine and Philosophy* 33, no. 6 (December 2008).

Campbell, A. G. M. "Quality of Life as a Decision-Making Criterion I." In *Ethics in Perinatology,* edited by Amnon Goldworth, William Silverman, David K. Stevenson, Ernle W. D. Young, and Rodney Rivers, 82-103. New York: Oxford University Press, 1995.

Campbell, A. G. M., and R. S. Duff. "Authors' Response to Richard Sherlock's Commentary." *Journal of Medical Ethics: The Journal of the Institute of Medical Ethics* 5 (Spring 1979): 141-42.

Catholic Health Association of the United States. "Continuing the Commitment: A Pathway to Health Care Reform" (April 2000).

Centers for Disease Control and Prevention. "Hospital Stays, Hospital Charges, and In-Hospital Deaths among Infants with Selected Birth Defects — United States, 2003." (2007).

Centers for Medicare and Medicaid Services. http://www.cms.hhs.gov/home/medicaid.asp (accessed June 23, 2008).

Christakis, D. A. "Continuity and Quality of Care for Children with Diabetes Who Are Covered by Medicaid." *Ambulatory Pediatrics* 1 (2001).

Clark, Peter A. *To Treat or Not to Treat: The Ethical Methodology of Richard A. McCormick, S.J., as Applied to Treatment Decisions for Handicapped Newborns.* Omaha: Creighton University Press, 2003.

Cohen, Andrew I., and Christopher Heath Wellman. *Contemporary Debates in Applied Ethics.* Contemporary Debates in Philosophy, vol. 3. Malden, Mass.: Blackwell, 2005.

Congregatio pro Doctrina Fidei. *Declaration on Euthanasia.* Washington, D.C.: Publications Office, United States Catholic Conference, 1980.

Curie, Janet, and Jeffrey Grogger. "Medicaid Expansions and Welfare Contractions: Offsetting Effects on Maternal Behavior and Infant Health." *Journal of Health Economics* 21 (2002): 313-35.

Curran, Charles E. *Catholic Social Teaching, 1891-Present: A Historical, Theological, and Ethical Analysis.* Moral Traditions Series. Washington, D.C.: Georgetown University Press, 2002.

Cuttini, Marina. *Ethical Issues in Neonatal Intensive Care and Physicians' Practices: A European Perspective.* Oslo: Scandinavian University Press, 2006.

Dahlburg, John Thor. "Where Killing Baby Girls Is 'No Big Sin.'" *Toronto Star,* February 28, 1994.

Damme, Catherine. "Infanticide: The Worth of an Infant under Law." *Medical History* 22 (1978): 1-24.

Degener, Theresia, and Yolan Koster-Dreese. "Human Rights and Disabled Persons: Essays and Relevant Human Rights Instruments." *International Studies in Human Rights* 40 (1995).

DeMone, J. A., P. C. Gonzalez, K. Gauvreau, G. E. Piercey, and K. J. Jenkins. "Risk of Death for Medicaid Recipients Undergoing Congenital Heart Surgery." *Pediatric Cardiology* 24, no. 2 (March 24, 2003).

Dombrowski, Daniel A., and Robert Deltete. *A Brief, Liberal, Catholic Defense of Abortion.* Champaign: University of Illinois Press, 2007.

Dorscheidt, J. H. M. *Levensbeeindiging Bij Gehandicapte Pasgeborenen: Strijdig Met Het Non-Discriminatiebeginsel?* The Hague: SDU, 2006.

Duff, Raymond. "Counseling Families and Deciding Care of Severely Defective Children: A Way of Coping with 'Medical Vietnam.'" *Pediatrics* 67 (March 1981): 315-20.

Dworkin, Ronald. *Life's Dominion: An Argument about Abortion, Euthanasia, and Individual Freedom.* New York: Knopf, 1993.

Edemariam, Aida. "Against All Odds." *Guardian,* February 21, 2007. http://www.guardian.co.uk/medicine/story/0,,2017772,00.html (accessed September 14, 2007).

Elliott, Kevin. "An Ironic Reductio for a Pro-Life Argument: Hurlbut's Proposal for Stem Cell Research." *Bioethics* 21, no. 2 (2007): 98-113.

Engelhardt, H. Tristram. *The Foundations of Bioethics.* New York: Oxford University Press, 1986.

Engelhardt, H. Tristram, and Mark J. Cherry. *Allocating Scarce Medical Resources: Roman Catholic Perspectives.* Clinical Medical Ethics Series. Washington, D.C.: Georgetown University Press, 2002.

Families USA. "Unwilling Volunteers: Tennesseans Forced Out of Health Care." http://www.familiesusa.org/resources/publications/reports/tenncarereport.html (accessed October 16, 2007).

Fins, Joseph J. "The Rationing of Health Care: A Doctor's Dilemma." *Journal of Religion and Health* 32, no. 1 (Spring 1993): 9-20.

Fletcher, Joseph Francis. "Four Indicators of Humanhood: The Enquiry Matures." *Hastings Center Report* 4, no. 6 (1974): 4-7.

Fost, Norm. "Decisions regarding Treatment of Seriously Ill Newborns." *Journal of the American Medical Association* 281 (1999).

Freedman, Benjamin. "Case for Medical Care, Inefficient or Not." *Hastings Center Report* 7, no. 2 (April 1977): 31-39.

Frohock, Fred M. "Euthanasia and the Newborn: Conflicts regarding Saving Lives." *Ethics* 99, no. 3 (April 1989): 689.

Gleason, Christine. *Almost Home: Stories of Hope and the Human Spirit.* New York: Kaplan Publishing, 2009.

Gruber, Jonathan, and the National Bureau of Economic Research. *Medicaid.* NBER Working Paper Series, working paper no. 7829. Cambridge, Mass.: National Bureau of Economic Research, 2000.

Guillemin, Jeanne Harley, and Lynda Lytle Holmstrom. *Mixed Blessings: Intensive Care for Newborns.* New York: Oxford University Press, 1986.

Hack, Maureen. "Chronic Conditions, Functional Limitations, and Special Health Care Needs of School-Aged Children Born with Extremely Low-Birth-Weight in the 1990s." *Journal of the American Medical Association* 294 (2005).

Hadorn, David C. "The Oregon Priority-Setting Exercise: Quality of Life and Public Policy." *Hastings Center Report* 21 (1991).

Hanson, Mark J., and Daniel Callahan. *The Goals of Medicine: The Forgotten Issue in Health Care Reform.* Hastings Center Studies in Ethics. Washington, D.C.: Georgetown University Press, 1999.

Henderson, Mark. "Genetic Mapping of Babies by 2019 Will Transform Preventive Medicine." *Times,* February 9, 2009. http://www.timesonline.co.uk/tol/news/uk/science/article5689052.ece (accessed August 12, 2009).

Himes, Kenneth R. *101 Questions on Catholic Social Teaching.* Mahwah, N.J.: Paulist, 2001.

Himes, Kenneth R., and Lisa Cahill. *Modern Catholic Social Teaching: Commentaries and Interpretations.* Washington, D.C.: Georgetown University Press, 2005.

"Indian Gov't to Raise Bandoned Girls." Associated Press. http://abcnews.go.com/Health/wireStory?id=2884808&CMP=OTC-RSSFeeds0312 (accessed March 13, 2007).

Intrator, Orna. "Effect of State Medicaid Reimbursement Rates on Hospitalizations from Nursing Homes." *Journal of the American Geriatrics Society* 52 (2004).

Jacobs, L. "The Oregon Health Plan and the Political Paradox of Rationing: What Advocates and Critics Have Claimed and What Oregon Did." *Journal of Health Policy, Politics and Law* 24 (1999).

John XXIII. *Mater et Magistra.* New York: Paulist, 1961.

John Paul II. *Centesimus Annus.* Washington, D.C.: Office for Publishing and Promotion Services, United States Catholic Conference, 1991.

———. *Sollicitudo Rei Socialis.* Washington, D.C.: Office of Publishing and Promotion Services, United States Catholic Conference, 1988.

Johnson, Paul. "Selective Nontreatment and Spina Bifida: A Case Study in Ethical Theory and Application." *Bioethics Quarterly* 3 (Summer 1981): 91-111.

———. "Selective Nontreatment of Defective Newborns: An Ethical Analysis." In *On Moral Medicine: Theological Perspectives in Medical Ethics,* edited by Stephen E. Lammers and Allen Verhey, 494-502. 1st ed. Grand Rapids: Eerdmans, 1987.

Karlekar, Malavika. "The Girl Child in India: Does She Have Any Rights?" *Canadian Woman Studies* (March 1995).

Kilner, John F. "A Moral Allocation of Scarce Lifesaving Medical Resources." *Journal of Religious Ethics* 9, no. 2 (Fall 1981): 245-85.

Kuhse, Helga, and Peter Singer. "Hard Choices: Ethical Questions Raised by the Birth of Handicapped Infants." In *Ethics on the Frontiers of Human Existence,* edited by Paul Badham. New York: Paragon House, 1992.

———. *Should the Baby Live? The Problem of Handicapped Infants.* Studies in Bioethics. Oxford and New York: Oxford University Press, 1985.

———, eds. *Bioethics: An Anthology.* 2nd ed. Blackwell Philosophy Anthologies, vol. 25. Malden, Mass., and Oxford: Blackwell, 2006.

Kumar, Sampath. "India Rights Campaign for Infanticide Mothers." BBC

News, July 17, 2003. http://news.bbc.co.uk/2/hi/south_asia/3071747.stm (accessed March 13, 2007).

LaCugna, Catherine Mowry. *God for Us: The Trinity and Christian Life.* San Francisco: HarperSanFrancisco, 1991.

Ladd, John. *Ethical Issues Relating to Life and Death.* Oxford: Oxford University Press, 1979.

Lammers, Stephen E., and Allen Verhey. *On Moral Medicine: Theological Perspectives in Medical Ethics.* Grand Rapids: Eerdmans, 1987.

Landon, Bruce E., Eric C. Schneider, Sharon-Lise T. Normand, Sarah Hudson Scholle, L. Gregory Pawlson, and Arnold M. Epstein. "Quality of Care in Medicaid Managed Care and Commercial Health Plans." *Journal of the American Medical Association* 298, no. 14 (October 10, 2007): 1674-81.

Lantos, John D. *Resource Allocation in Neonatal and Medical ICUs: Epidemiology and Rationing at the Extremes of Life.* Vol. 156. [New York]: American Lung Association, 1997.

Lantos, John D., and William Meadow. *Neonatal Bioethics: The Moral Challenges of Medical Innovation.* Baltimore: Johns Hopkins University Press, 2006.

La Pine, Timothy R., J. Craig Jackson, and F. C. Bennett. "Outcome of Infants Weighing Less Than 800 Grams at Birth: 15 Years' Experience." *Pediatrics* 96 (1995).

Laurance, Jeremy. "Critics Condemn '23-Week' Premature Baby Ban." *Independent,* November 16, 2006. http://news.independent.co.uk/uk/health_medical/article1987614.ece (accessed January 27, 2007).

Lauritzen, Paul, ed. *Cloning and the Future of Human Embryo Research.* Oxford and New York: Oxford University Press, 2001.

Leo XIII. *Immortale Dei.* New York: Paulist, 1941.

————. *Rerum Novarum.* New York: Paulist, 1900.

Leuthner, Steven R. *Fetal Palliative Care.* Vol. 31. Philadelphia: Elsevier, 2004.

Lizza, John P. *Persons, Humanity, and the Definition of Death.* Baltimore: Johns Hopkins University Press, 2006.

Lucas, Fred. "White House Vows No Rationing in Health Care Reform Package." CNS News, June 3, 2009. http://www.cnsnews.com/Public/Content/article.aspx?RsrcID=49010 (accessed June 27, 2009).

Marquis, Don. "Why Abortion Is Immoral." *Journal of Philosophy* 86 (1989): 183-202.

Matthews, Eric, and Michael Menlowe. *Philosophy and Health Care.* Avebury Series in Philosophy. Aldershot, England, and Brookfield, Vt.: Avebury, 1992.

McCarthy, Robert. "Triage for the Poor in Oregon — Recasting of Medicaid Payment Disorder Ranking." *Business and Health* (April 1991).

McCartney, James. "Issues in Death and Dying." In *Moral Theology: Challenges for the Future.* Mahwah, N.J.: Paulist, 2003.

McCormick, Richard A. "The Best Interests of the Baby." *Second Opinion* 2 (July 1986): 18-25.

———. *Corrective Vision: Explorations in Moral Theology.* Kansas City, Mo.: Sheed and Ward, 1994.

———. *The Critical Calling: Reflections on Moral Dilemmas since Vatican II.* Washington, D.C.: Georgetown University Press, 1989.

———. "Experimentation in Children: Sharing in Sociality." *Hastings Center Report* 6 (December 1976): 41-46.

———. *Health and Medicine in the Catholic Tradition: Tradition in Transition.* New York: Crossroad, 1984.

———. *How Brave a New World? Dilemmas in Bioethics.* 1st ed. Garden City, N.Y.: Doubleday, 1981.

———. "Quality of Life, the Sanctity of Life." *Hastings Center Report* 8 (Fall 1978): 30-36.

———. "The Preservation of Life." *Linacre Quarterly* 43 (May 1976): 94-100.

———. "To Save or Let Die: The Dilemma of Modern Medicine." *Journal of the American Medical Association* 229 (July 8, 1974): 172-76.

McCormick, Richard A., and John Paris. "Saving Defective Infants: Options for Life or Death." *America,* April 23, 1983, 313-17.

McDonough, Mary Joan. *Can a Health Care Market Be Moral? A Catholic Vision.* Washington, D.C.: Georgetown University Press, 2007.

McInerney, Peter K. "Does a Fetus Already Have a Future-Like-Ours?" *Journal of Philosophy* 87, no. 5 (May 1990): 264-68.

Meadow, William, and John Lantos. "Changes in Mortality for Extremely Low Birth Weight Infants in the 1990s: Implications for Treatment Decisions and Resource Use." *Pediatrics* 113 (2004).

"Medicaid Squeeze." *Online Newshour,* March 2, 2005. http://www.pbs.org/newshour/bb/health/jan-june05/medicaid_3-02.html (accessed October 16, 2007).

Mercurio, M. R. "Parental Authority and the Patient's Best Interest." *Journal of Perinatology* 26 (2006): 452-57.

Merkens, Mark J., and Michael J. Garland. "The Oregon Health Plan and the Ethics of Care for Marginally Viable Newborns." *Journal of Clinical Ethics* 12 (Fall 2001): 266-73.

Midgley, Mary. *Animals and Why They Matter.* Athens: University of Georgia Press, 1984.

Miller, Geoffrey. *Extreme Prematurity: Practices, Bioethics, and the Law.* Cambridge and New York: Cambridge University Press, 2007.

Morse, Steven B., Samuel S. Wu, Changxing Ma, Mario Ariet, Michael Resnick, and Jeffrey Roth. "Racial and Gender Differences in the Viability of Extremely Low Birth Weight Infants: A Population-Based Study" (2006).

National Conference of Catholic Bishops. *Economic Justice for All: Pastoral Letter on Catholic Social Teaching and the U.S. Economy.* Vol. 101. Washington, D.C.: Office of Publishing and Promotion Services, United States Catholic Conference, 1986.

————. "U.S. Bishops' Pastoral Letter on Healthcare." (1981).

National Conference of Catholic Bishops: Committee for Pro-Life Activities and American Jewish Congress. "Treatment of Handicapped Newborns." (July 26, 1985).

"Nearly 5 Babies Killed Weekly, FBI Data Show." CNN, June 27, 1997. http://www.cnn.com/US/9706/27/killed.babies/index.html (accessed March 13, 2007).

Nuffield Council on Bioethics. "Critical Care Decisions in Fetal and Neonatal Medicine." (2006).

O'Rourke, Kevin D., and Philip Boyle. *Medical Ethics: Sources of Catholic Teachings.* 3rd ed. Washington, D.C.: Georgetown University Press, 1999.

Panicola, Michael R. "Quality of Life and the Critically Ill Newborn: Life and Death Decision Making in the Neonatal Context." Ph.D. diss., Saint Louis University, 2000.

Paris, John. "Letter to the Editors: Handicapped Infants and Their Families." *Law, Medicine and Healthcare* 11 (October 1983): 231.

————. "Parental Discretion in Refusal of Treatment for Newborns." *Clinics in Perinatology* 23 (September 1996): 573-81.

Paris, John, and Richard McCormick. "The Catholic Tradition on the Use of Nutrition and Fluids." *America,* May 2, 1987, 356-61.

Paul VI. *Octogesima Adveniens.* New York: Paulist, 1971.

————. *Populorum Progressio.* New York: Paulist, 1967.

Pennsylvania Catholic Bishops. *Nutrition and Hydration: Moral Considerations.* (1999).

Perrett, Roy W. "Taking Life and the Argument from Potentiality." *Midwest Studies in Philosophy* 24 (2000): 186-98.

Pinker, Steven. "Why They Kill Their Newborns." *New York Times,* November 2, 1997.

Pius XI. *Divini Redemptoris.* New York: Paulist, 1930.

————. *Quadragesimo Anno.* Washington, D.C.: National Catholic Welfare Conference, 1942.

Pius XII. "Prolongation of Life." *Pope Speaks* 4 (1958): 395-96.

Pontificium Consilium de Iustitia et Pace. *Compendium of the Social Doctrine of the Church.* Dublin: Veritas, 2005.

President's Commission for the Study of Ethical Problems in Medicine and Biomedical and Behavioral Research. *Deciding to Forego Life-Sustaining Treatment: A Report on the Ethical, Medical, and Legal Issues in Treatment Decisions.*

Washington, D.C.: President's Commission for the Study of Ethical Problems in Medicine and Biomedical and Behavioral Research, 1983.

Profit, Jochen. "Neonatal Intensive Care Unit Census Influences Discharge of Moderately Preterm Infants." *Pediatrics* (2007).

Ramsey, Paul. "Children as Research Subjects: A Reply." *Hastings Center Report* 7 (April 1977): 40-42.

————. "Enforcement of Morals: Nontherapeutic Research on Children." *Hastings Center Report* 6 (August 1976): 21-29.

————. *Ethics at the Edges of Life: Medical and Legal Intersections.* New Haven: Yale University Press, 1978.

————. *The Patient as Person: Explorations in Medical Ethics.* Lyman Beecher Lectures at Yale University. New Haven: Yale University Press, 1970.

————. "The Sanctity of Life — in the First of It." *Dublin Review* 511 (Spring 1967): 3-23.

Reichlin, Massimo. "The Argument from Potential: A Reappraisal." *Bioethics* 11, no. 1 (January 1997): 1-23.

Salo, Mikko A. "Triage in Social Policy." *Acta Philosophica Fennica* 68 (2001): 155-71.

Schmeida, Mary, Ramona McNeal, and Kathleen Hale. "Facing Medicaid Budget Shortfall in 2006: State Context Influences Government Health Service Cut-Backs." Paper presented at the annual meeting of the American Political Science Association, Philadelphia, August 31, 2006.

Schmitt, Susan K. "Costs of Newborn Care in California: A Population-Based Study." *Pediatrics* 117 (2006).

Schwartz, Lita Linzer, and Natalie Isser. *Endangered Children: Neonaticide, Infanticide, Filicide.* Pacific Institute Series on Forensic Psychology. Boca Raton, Fla.: CRC Press, 2000.

Sears, Neal. "Outrage as Church Calls for Severely Disabled Babies to Be Killed at Birth." *MailOnline,* November 12, 2006. http://www.dailymail.co.uk/pages/live/articles/news/news.html?in_article_id=416003&in_page_id=1770 (accessed January 27, 2007).

Shaw, Anthony. "Defining the Quality of Life." *Hastings Center Report* 7, no. 5 (October 1977): 11.

Shearer, M. H. "The Economics of Intensive-Care for the Full-Term Newborn." *Birth* 7, no. 4 (1980).

Shelp, Earl E. *Born to Die? Deciding the Fate of Critically Ill Newborns.* New York: Free Press; London: Collier Macmillan, 1986.

Silverman, W. A. "Mismatched Attitudes about Neonatal Death." *Hastings Center Report* 11, no. 6 (December 1981): 12-16.

————. "Overtreatment of Neonates? A Personal Retrospective." *Pediatrics* 90 (1992).

Singer, Peter. *Practical Ethics.* 2nd ed. Cambridge and New York: Cambridge University Press, 1993.

————. *Rethinking Life and Death: The Collapse of Our Traditional Ethics.* New York: St. Martin's Griffin, 1996.

————. "Why We Must Ration Health Care." *New York Times Magazine,* July 15, 2009. http://www.nytimes.com/2009/07/19/magazine/19healthcare-t.html (accessed August 10, 2009).

Singh, Jaideep. "Resuscitation in the 'Gray Zone' of Viability: Determining Physician Preferences and Predicting Infant Outcomes." *Pediatrics* 120 (2007).

Soranus. *Gynecology.* Johns Hopkins University. Institute of the History of Medicine. Publications. Second Series. Texts and Documents. Baltimore: Johns Hopkins University Press, 1956.

Sparks, Richard C. *To Treat or Not to Treat: Bioethics and the Handicapped Newborn.* New York: Paulist, 1988.

Stanley, J. M. *The Appleton Consensus: Suggested International Guidelines for Decisions to Forego Medical Treatment.* Vol. 15. London: British Medical Association, 1989.

Stark, Rodney. *The Rise of Christianity: A Sociologist Reconsiders History.* Princeton: Princeton University Press, 1996.

Steinbock, Bonnie. "Why Most Abortions Are Not Wrong." *Advances in Bioethics* 5 (1999): 245-67.

Stolz, J. W. "Restricting Access to Neonatal Intensive Care: Effect on Mortality and Economic Savings." *Pediatrics* 101 (1998).

Synodus Episcoporum. *The Synodal Document on the Justice in the World.* Boston: St. Paul Editions, 1971.

Tanner, Lindsey. "Who Should MDs Let Die in a Pandemic?" *Boston Globe,* May 5, 2008.

Templeton, Sarah-Kate. "Doctors: Let Us Kill Disabled Babies." *Times Online,* November 5, 2006. http://www.timesonline.co.uk/tol/news/uk/article 625477.ece (accessed April 4, 2007).

Tooley, Michael. *Abortion and Infanticide.* Oxford: Clarendon; New York: Oxford University Press, 1983.

Troyer, Jennifer L. "Examining Differences in Death Rates for Medicaid and Non-Medicaid Nursing Home Residents." *Medical Care* 42 (2004).

Tyson, Jon E., Nehal A. Parikh, John Langer, Charles Green, and Rosemary D. Higgins. "Intensive Care for Extreme Prematurity — Moving beyond Gestational Age." *New England Journal of Medicine* 358 (April 2008).

United Nations General Assembly. "Convention of the Rights of Persons with Disabilities." (December 6, 2006). http://www.un.org/esa/socdev/enable/rights/convtexte.htm (accessed September 15, 2007).

United States Catholic Conference of Bishops. "Nutrition and Hydration: Moral and Pastoral Reflections." *Origins Online* 21, no. 44 (1992).

United States Equal Employment Opportunity Commission. "Section 902: Definition of the Term Disability." http://www.eeoc.gov/policy/docs/902cm.html (accessed September 15, 2007).

Urban Institute. "Uninsured and Dying Because of It." http://www.urban.org/UploadedPDF/411588_uninsured_dying.pdf (accessed August 6, 2008).

Vatican Council II. *Pastoral Constitution on the Church in the Modern World: Gaudium et Spes, December 7, 1965.* Washington, D.C.: National Catholic Welfare Conference, 1976.

Verhagen, E., and P. J. Sauer. "The Groningen Protocol — Euthanasia in Severely Ill Newborns." *New England Journal of Medicine* 352, no. 10 (March 10, 2005): 959-62.

Walter, James J. "Termination of Medical Treatment: The Setting of Moral Limits from Infancy to Old Age." *Religious Studies Review* 16 (October 1990): 302-7.

Walter, James J., and Thomas A. Shannon. *Quality of Life: The New Medical Dilemma.* New York: Paulist, 1990.

Weigert, Kathleen Maas, and Alexia K. Kelley. *Living the Catholic Social Tradition: Cases and Commentary.* Lanham, Md.: Rowman and Littlefield, 2005.

Werpehowski, William, and Stephen D. Crocco, eds. *The Essential Paul Ramsey.* New Haven: Yale University Press, 1994.

Whitmore, Todd David. "Catholic Social Teaching: A Synthesis." January 14, 2004.

Wolfberg, Adam. "Extreme Preemies." *Boston Globe,* April 27, 2008.

"World Death Rate Is Holding Steady at 100%." *Onion,* January 22, 1997. http://www.theonion.com/articles/world-death-rate-holding-steady-at-100-percent,1670/ (accessed June 27, 2009).

# Index